W9-BLY-695

GETTING IN SHAPE

WORKOUT PROGRAMS
FOR MEN AND WOMEN

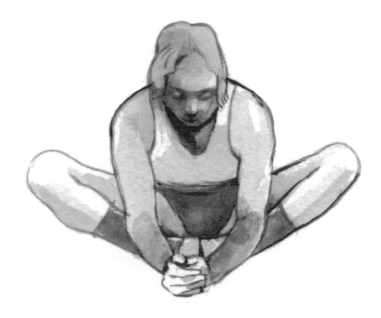

Bob Anderson

Bill Pearl

Edmund R. Burke, Ph.D.

Illustrated by Jean Anderson

Shelter Publications, Inc.
Bolinas, California

Copyright © 1994 by Shelter Publications, Inc.

All rights reserved. No part of this publication may be reproduced or transmitted in any form or by any means, electronic of mechanical, including photocopy, recording, computer scanning or any information and retrieval system without the written permission of the publisher. *Exception:* Readers who purchase this book may make a photocopy of any of the programs in the book for their own personal use.

Distibuted in the United States by Publishers Group West and in Canada by Publishers Group West Canada.

LIBRARY OF CONGRESS CATALOGING-IN-PUBLICATION DATA

Anderson, Bob, 1945–
     Getting in shape : workout programs for men and women / Bob Anderson, Bill Pearl,
  Edmund R. Burke
        p.   cm.
     Includes bibliographical references and index.
     ISBN 0–936070–16–1 : $14.95.
     1. Physical fitness. 2. Exercise. I. Pearl, Bill, 1930–.   II. Burke, Ed, 1949–.
  III. Title.
  GV481.A45   1994   94–21737
  613.7–dc20   CIP

We are grateful to the following publishers for permission to reprint portions of previously published material:

Reed Consumer Books/Mitchell Beazley, London, U. K. for quote on p. 112 from *The Rand McNally Atlas of the Body* ©1980

Rodale's *Food and Nutrition* Magazine for "Eight Suggestions for Cutting Your Oil Bill" on p. 131

Body Bulletin Magazine (Feb. '91 issue) for "The Top 15 Personal Cancer-Prevention Measures" on p. 152

Fitness Cycling Magazine for photos used as basis for drawings on p. 158, "Wrist Exercises for Carpal Tunnel Syndrome"

Houghton Mifflin Company for chart on p. 180 from *The New Fit or Fat.* ©1977, 1978, 1991 by Covert Bailey. Reprinted by permission of Houghton Mifflin Co. All rights reserved.

We are also grateful to Dr. Steven N. Blair and his book *Living with Exercise* (see p. 200) for inspiration for "History of Human Fitness" on p. 110.

  6 7 8 9 — 03 02 01 00
(Lowest digits indicate number and year of this printing.)

Printed in the United States of America

Medical Warning: Please get a physical before trying any of the programs in this book, especially if you are overweight, have not exercised for a while, have had any health problems or if there is any family history of health problems.

Additional copies of this book may be purchased at your favorite bookstore, or by sending $14.95 plus $3.95 shipping and handling to:

     Shelter Publications, Inc.
     P. O. Box 279
     Bolinas, California 94924
     415-868-0280
     Orders, toll-free: 1-800-307-0131
     Email: shelter@shelterpub.com

Visit Our Website
SHELTER ONLINE
http://www.shelterpub.com

CONTENTS

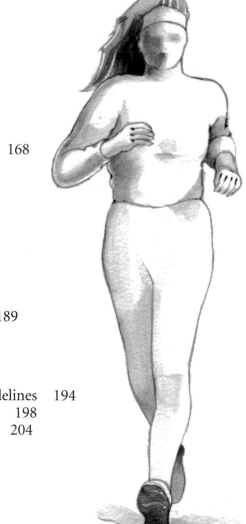

A BRIEF INTRODUCTION

Among the three of us, we have spent a total of some 90 years working in three different fields of physical activity:

- Bob in stretching
- Bill in weight training
- Ed in aerobic exercise

We've worked with many thousands of people, all the way from "one-on-ones" to lectures and workshops for crowds.

We've watched the fads come and go.

We think we've learned what works — and what does not.

We've seen that the exercise programs and "fitness prescriptions" of the last two decades have not worked for most people. For one thing, the standards have been too high for the average person. (Less than 10% of Americans now exercise enough to get cardiorespiratory health benefits.)

We've also seen a growing appreciation over the past few years for the value of "moderate" exercise. Something one can stick with for a lifetime.

We believe that what's needed in this day and age are structured, balanced workout programs which:

- are not too extreme
- are mainly graphic
- let you choose your level of commitment
- will fit within your busy schedule

So we've combined our experience to produce *Getting In Shape.*

Using this book will start you on a gradual, steady path that will lead to a lifetime of:

- better cardiovascular health
- greater strength
- improved flexibility

Give it a try.

Be relaxed, have fun.

Bob Anderson   *Bill Pearl*   *Edmund R. Burke*

PART ONE

ACTION

1   THE BASICS

Putting it simply, you will do three basic things:

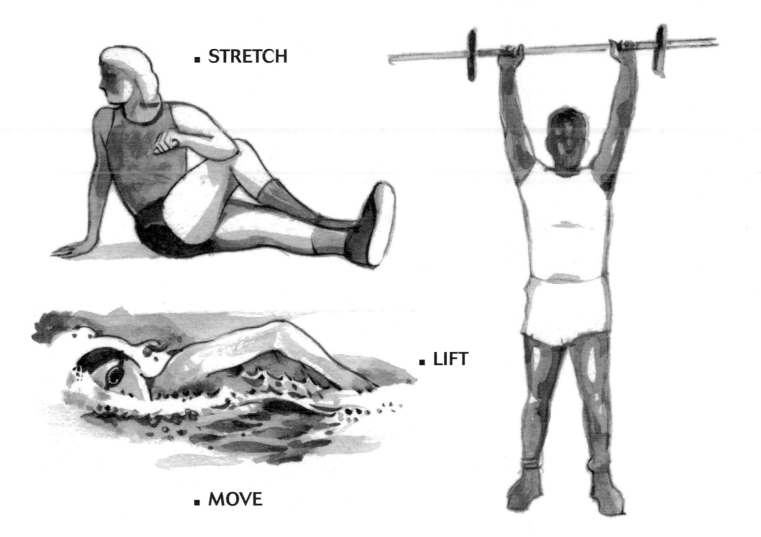

. STRETCH

. LIFT

. MOVE

- **Stretching** will make you more *flexible*.

- **Lifting** will make you *stronger*.

- **Moving** will strengthen your *heart* and *lungs* and improve *circulation*.

GETTING A PHYSICAL

If you are over 35 or have been inactive for a few years, see your physician before beginning any exercise program. This is especially important if your family has a history of heart disease, high blood pressure, high cholesterol, diabetes, arthritis, obesity, cigarette smoking, or other health conditions.

However, if neither you nor your family has had these problems, you can probably start these programs without consulting a doctor. These programs are moderate and not extremely vigorous.

If you have any doubts whatsoever, consult your physician.

HOW TO USE THIS BOOK

Getting in Shape is divided into two sections:

- Part One is **Action**. It contains all the programs, exercises, and instructions — what to do and how to do it *(pages 6 to 108)*.

- Part Two is **Thought**. This contains information and general and specific guidelines on health and fitness.

The exercise programs in this book are easy to use. They are primarily visual and are displayed on one- or two-page spreads for easy reference. You can photocopy a program and take it with you wherever you work out.

Before you begin, read the general principles which follow on how to stretch, how to lift, and how to move. Following these guidelines will facilitate your progress. Exercising the right way gives the best payback on the time and effort you invest.

The first time you perform a program, follow the instructions carefully for each stretch or exercise. (There are page references to instructions for each stretch and exercise in all programs.) Look at the instructions each time you work out, until you know them by heart. After that, simply look at the drawings in the programs.

HOW TO STRETCH

Stretching is simple. But there is a right way and a wrong way to stretch. The right way is to stretch slowly, be relaxed, and focus on the muscles being stretched. The wrong way (practiced by many) is to bounce, or to push the stretch to the point of pain or beyond; these methods can do more harm than good.

THE EASY STRETCH

Stretch to the point where you feel a *mild tension,* then relax as you hold the stretch for 5 to 15 seconds. NO BOUNCING! The feeling of tension should ease as you hold the stretch. If it doesn't, ease off slightly until things feel comfortable. The easy stretch reduces muscular tightness and readies the muscles for the developmental stretch.

THE DEVELOPMENTAL STRETCH

Move slowly into the developmental stretch, a fraction of an inch farther, until you feel mild tension, and hold it for 5 to 15 seconds. No bouncing. Again, the tension should diminish. If not, ease off.

THE ONE-PHASE STRETCH

Doing just the easy stretch will release tension and make you feel better. It's valuable even without the developmental stretch. It helps you maintain your current flexibility.

BREATHE

Breathe slowly and naturally. Do not hold your breath while stretching.

6

RELAX

Keep your hands, feet, shoulders, and jaw relaxed as you stretch. Tension there will hinder your stretching.

THE STRETCH REFLEX

Whenever you stretch muscle fibers too far (either by bouncing or pushing too far), a nerve reflex signals the muscles to contract. This *stretch reflex* is one of the body's automatic defense mechanisms and keeps the muscles from being injured. When you overdo it, you tighten the very muscles you're trying to stretch.

A word of caution: pushing a stretch too far or bouncing can strain the muscles and activate the stretch reflex. If you stretch too far, you may cause microscopic damage to the muscle fibers. These small muscle tears lead to formation of scar tissue, with a gradual loss of elasticity.

NO PAIN, NO GAIN?

Pain is a sign something is *wrong* in stretching. Pay attention to it and back off! Most stretching injuries have come from people pushing too far or too fast.

WHAT'S THE RIGHT FEELING?

It should feel mild, not intense. It should feel like you can hold it indefinitely. We all have different levels of flexibility; don't compare yourself with others. Stretching isn't a contest. Everyone is different.

HOW TO LIFT

Proper technique will help you get the most out of weightlifting, and will help prevent injuries.

REPS AND SETS

For each exercise in the Programs, we indicate *reps* and *sets*.

- *Rep* is short for repetition, or one complete movement (up and down or back and forth), of an exercise. Completion of a rep means you return to starting position.

- A *set* is a fixed number of reps.

HOW MUCH WEIGHT?

Use enough weight so you can complete the prescribed sets and reps fairly comfortably, but the *last rep should feel difficult*. This will give your muscles the right amount of resistance (weight) to start building them stronger, but not so much that you injure yourself. As you make progress, and the last rep of the set starts feeling easy, increase the weight — using the same principle.

PROPER POSITION

In a standing position, keep your feet a little wider than shoulder-width apart and balanced fore and aft. Keep head and neck straight. Many lifting injuries are caused by twisting the head, neck, or trunk. Leverage is not as good and muscle injuries often occur when the spine is twisted. Always go through the full range of motion with each exercise.

When using a bench, try to keep your legs positioned at the sides and your feet flat on the floor. If the bench is too tall, place your feet on the end with your knees bent. Raise and lower the weight with complete control, making a definite pause with each rep. Keep your head on the bench and do not arch your back too sharply or raise your hips off the bench.

BREATHING

Inhale at the start of the lift, *momentarily* hold your breath during the most difficult part, and exhale as you finish. Breathe in and out through the nose *and* mouth. Do *not* hold your breath.

- Use collars on barbells. It's tempting to save time by leaving off collars, but the weights can slip off the end and cause injury.

- Use proper positions. Study the drawings.

- Don't jerk or twist when lifting. These movements increase stress and can cause injuries.

DAY OF REST

This simple principle is part of *progressive resistance training*. Do not lift weights two days in a row. A 24-hour rest period allows the muscles you've been working to adapt to the increased load. In weight training, you stress or "overload" the muscle beyond the demands of previous activity. When this is followed by a rest period, the muscles rebuild with greater strength.

**NOTICE HOW
YOU FEEL**

On your day of rest, spend some time noticing the benefits of your training, a new and pleasant sensation of physical awareness. Almost immediately you'll feel firmer, improved muscle tone. You'll have more energy and a strong sense of how good it feels to move and be more active.

If you don't have that good feeling, you need to train harder. Increase the weights, add a few more reps to each set, or move ahead to the next level in the Programs. On the other hand, if you feel excessively sore or stiff, cut back some. You can expect a little discomfort as your muscles and joints adapt, but you should not feel pain.

HOW TO MOVE

On pages 64–73 are some ideas for more effective walking, cycling, swimming, or running. Remember, you are not limited to these activities: you needn't always put on a sweatsuit and pound down the pavement to improve your heart and lungs. There's tennis, golf, softball, or productive activities like working in the garden, cleaning the house, washing the car — anything that gets you moving and gets your heart pumping harder.

Checking your heart rate will tell you how hard you're working your heart. It's especially important if you haven't exercised for a while. Do this when you start exercising, whether with typical athletic activities, such as walking, running, cycling, or swimming, or working in the garden, shoveling snow, or dancing.

HEART RATE

See page 117 for specific directions on how to check your heart rate.

- *The Program Before the Program:* Don't worry about heart rate if you are following these preliminary programs, since you will be exercising at such a moderate level. Just don't get uncomfortably out of breath.

- *Basic Programs 1–5:* Here, you'll want to start checking your heart rate so you understand how your heart responds to exercise. Exercise at a *comfortable* rate, checking your pulse and comparing it to your maximum heart rate. Don't worry about percentages at first.

- *After you get in better shape:* A reasonable zone would be 50% of maximum or higher.

PERCEIVED EXERTION METHOD

This is the intuitive, rather than scientific method. After you check your pulse for a while, you'll be able to tell from your own breathing how hard you're working. You'll get a sense when you're moving fast enough to get a training effect. For example, if you decide to exercise at 50% of your maximum heart rate, take your pulse and concentrate on how this level *feels.* Many factors will go into this, such as how you feel that day, the condition you're in, the heat, headwinds, etc., all of which can be measured by how out-of-breath you are. After you do this for a while, you'll be able to make a close-enough guess of a 50% rate without taking your pulse or counting.

LONGER WORKOUT/LOWER INTENSITY

Many people prefer longer, slower workouts. (By "longer" we're referring to the times indicated in the Programs.) You might enjoy longer, more relaxed workouts, at a lower pulse rate. The benefits can be the same. Feel free to experiment.

EFFECT OF MEDICATIONS ON HEART RATE

Certain types of medication do affect your heart rate; for example, the class of drugs known as beta blockers, often prescribed for high blood pressure or chest pains, lowers your heart rate. Many other medications affect heart rate (tranquilizers, diet and thyroid medications, bronchodilators, etc.), so if you are taking anything, check with your doctor. *(See pp. 165–167 on high blood pressure.)*

RULE OF THUMB

You should be able to carry on a conversation while exercising.

2 THE PROGRAMS

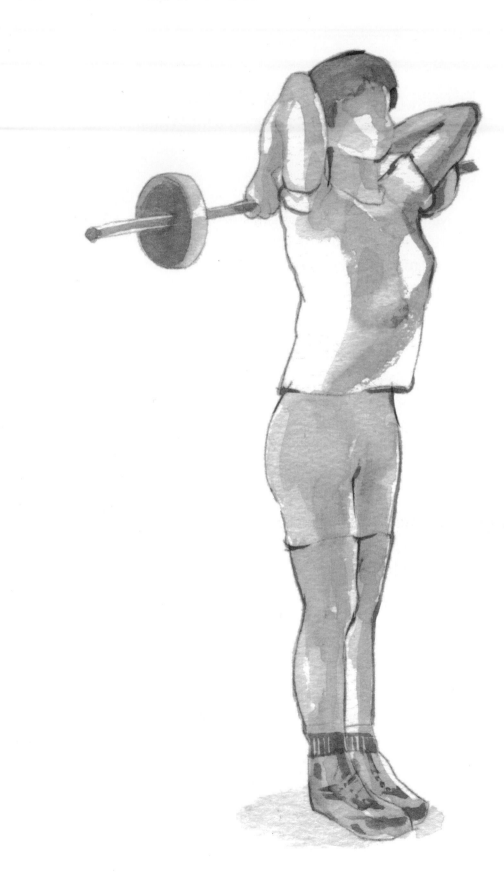

32 PROGRAMS PREVIEW

THE PROGRAM BEFORE THE PROGRAM – 3 PHASES

Start here if you:

- haven't exercised in some time
- are overweight
- are recovering from an illness or surgery
- for any reason have doubts about Basic Program 1

5 BASIC PROGRAMS

Skip ahead and look at Basic Program 1 (pp. 20–21) now.

Start here if you:

- feel in good enough shape, or
- have completed the Program Before the Program

16 SPECIAL PROGRAMS

These are for special situations.

At Work
- Desk Stretches
- On the Job
- The Busy Day

On the Road
- Airplane Stretches
- Hotel Room Workout

Stretch & Strengthen

Circuit Training
- Basic Circuit Training
- Super Circuit Training

Electronic Gym
- LifeCircuit Training
- LifeCircuit & Free Weights

Health Programs
- Arthritis
- Back Pain
- Carpal Tunnel Syndrome
- Weight Management

8 FINE TUNING PROGRAMS

These are overall body workout programs, each emphasizing a different body part.

- Abdominals
- Arms
- Back
- Buttocks
- Calves
- Chest
- Legs
- Shoulders

WARM UP AND COOL DOWN

FOR ALL PROGRAMS:

Your workouts will consist of 3 phases:

1. STRETCH & WARM UP

Stretching and warming up are two different things.

- Stretch gently before you warm up by doing the stretches shown in the program you are about to do. It gets the muscles ready for action. If you want, do a light circulation warmup before you stretch, such as a 1-minute walk with a big arm swing.

- Warm up by doing some of the exercise you are about to do, but at a lower intensity. Rule of thumb: break a light sweat.

2. EXERCISE

- Lift weights (follow the programs)

  AND/OR

- Move (get your heart rate up)

3. COOL DOWN & STRETCH

- Cool down by doing a scaled-down version of the main workout. Get your heart and muscles back down toward resting rate.

- Stretch after you cool down to prevent soreness and stiffness. You can do the same stretches *after* that you did *before*.

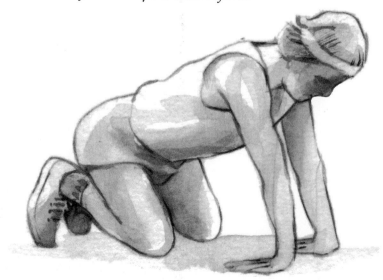

THE PROGRAM BEFORE THE PROGRAM

UP & MOVING

WHAT WILL THIS PROGRAM DO FOR ME?

Get you up and moving and in good enough shape for
Basic Programs 1 to 5.

WHO DOESN'T NEED TO FOLLOW THIS PROGRAM?

Look at Basic Program 1 on pp. 20–21. If you think you can follow it
easily, skip this section. You're in good enough shape to start the Basic
Programs. If you do start Basic Program 1 and it's too tough, come
back and start here. Be honest with yourself about where to begin. If
you try to do too much too soon, you may give up and quit. Setting
realistic goals and taking it slowly will enable you to succeed.

WHAT EQUIPMENT DO I NEED?

None (other than perhaps a pair of walking shoes). Here you are using
your body weight for the weight training exercises.

WHAT ABOUT HEART RATE?

- These exercises are so mild you don't need to check heart rate, as
  long as you don't overdo it.
- Keep it light.
- Take it easy. Be comfortable.
- Start slowly, especially with moving exercise. It's the only way you'll
  make steady progress.
- Don't push too far. You should be able to talk while exercising.

HOW DO I MOVE FROM ONE LEVEL TO ANOTHER?

- Stay on Level 1 until you feel ready for Level 2.
- Stay on Level 2 until you feel ready for Level 3.*

HOW MUCH TIME WILL THIS TAKE?

- Level 1 will take about 10 minutes a day.
- Level 2 will take about 15 minutes a day.
- Level 3 will take about 25 minutes a day.

*If you get to any one level and are satisfied with your level of fitness, stay on that level as long as you
care to. You will *maintain* whatever level of fitness you have already achieved.

PROGRAM BEFORE THE PROGRAM 1

Stretch every day. Lift OR Move on alternate days.

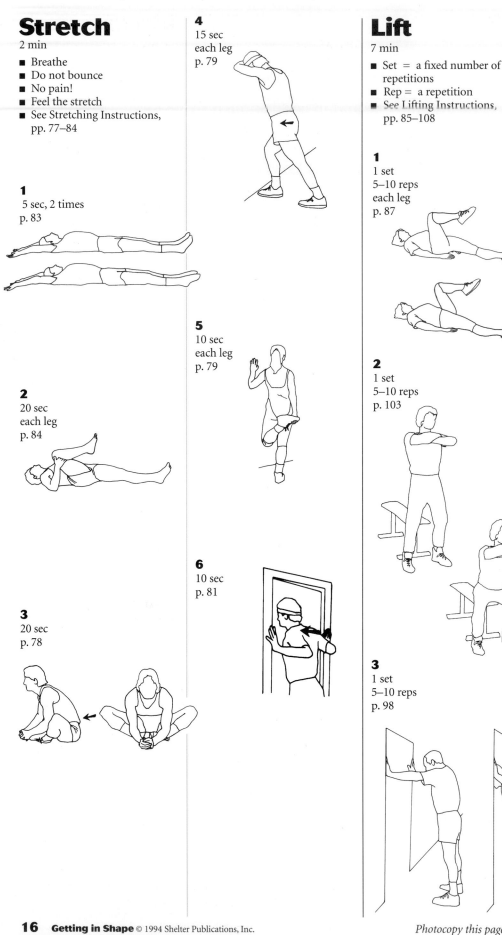

Stretch
2 min

- Breathe
- Do not bounce
- No pain!
- Feel the stretch
- See Stretching Instructions, pp. 77–84

1
5 sec, 2 times
p. 83

2
20 sec
each leg
p. 84

3
20 sec
p. 78

4
15 sec
each leg
p. 79

5
10 sec
each leg
p. 79

6
10 sec
p. 81

Lift
7 min

- Set = a fixed number of repetitions
- Rep = a repetition
- See Lifting Instructions, pp. 85–108

1
1 set
5–10 reps
each leg
p. 87

2
1 set
5–10 reps
p. 103

3
1 set
5–10 reps
p. 98

Move
6–8 min

Sit less. Change your habits:

- Take the stairs instead of the elevator
- Park farther away
- Sit instead of lying down
- Stand instead of sitting
- Move instead of standing
- See Moving Instructions, pp. 64–76

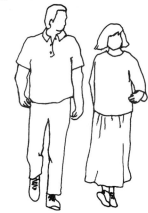

WALK
5 min whenever you can, several times a day.

OR
Do anything that gets you moving.

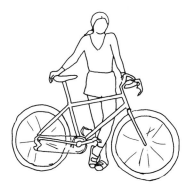

Photocopy this page and take it with you when you work out.

PROGRAM BEFORE THE PROGRAM 2

Stretch every day. Lift OR Move on alternate days.

Stretch
4 min
- Breathe easily
- Do not bounce
- No pain!
- Feel each stretch
- See Stretching Instructions, pp. 77–84

1
15 sec
p. 81

2
5 sec, 2 times
p. 81

3
10 sec
each side
p. 82

4
20 sec
each leg
p. 79

5
15 sec
each leg
p. 79

6
30 sec
p. 78

7
30 sec
each leg
p. 84

8
5 sec
each side
p. 83

Lift
13 min
- Set = a fixed number of repetitions
- Rep = a repetition
- See Lifting Instructions, pp. 85–108

1
1 set
5–10 reps
each leg
p. 87

2
1 set
5–10 reps
p. 86

3
1 set
10–12 reps
p. 103

4
1 set
5–10 reps
p. 96

5
1 set
10–12 reps
p. 98

6
1 set
5–10 reps
p. 91

Move
5–10 min
- See Moving Instructions, pp. 64–76

WALK
5 min
whenever
you can

OR

SWIM
10 min

Stop and rest whenever needed.

OR

DO YARDWORK OR HOUSEWORK
mow lawn, wash car, vacuum, etc.

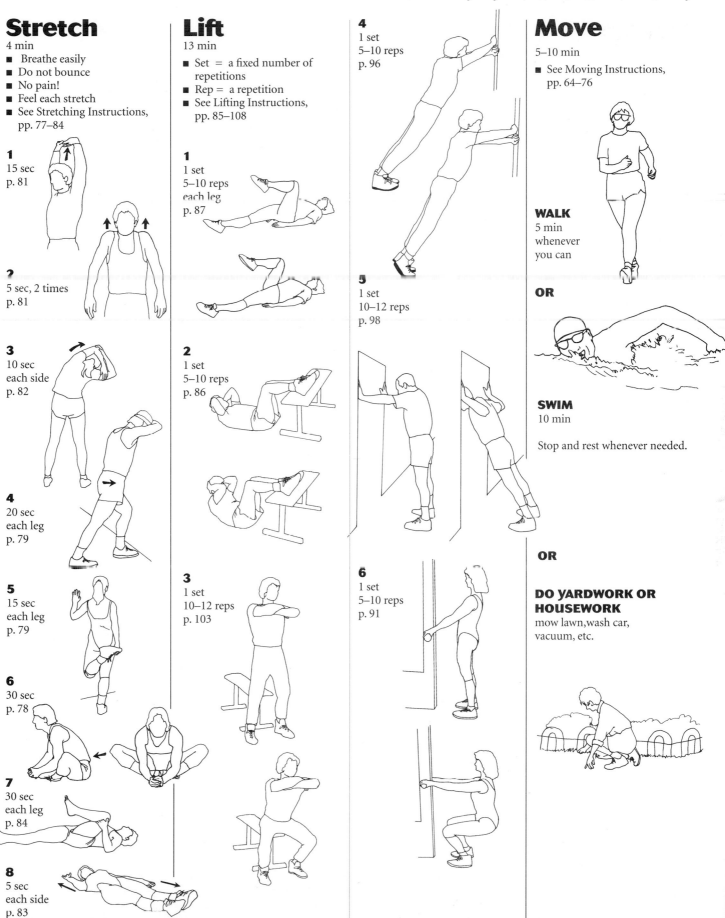

Photocopy this page and take it with you when you work out.

PROGRAM BEFORE THE PROGRAM 3

Stretch every day. Lift OR Move on alternate days.

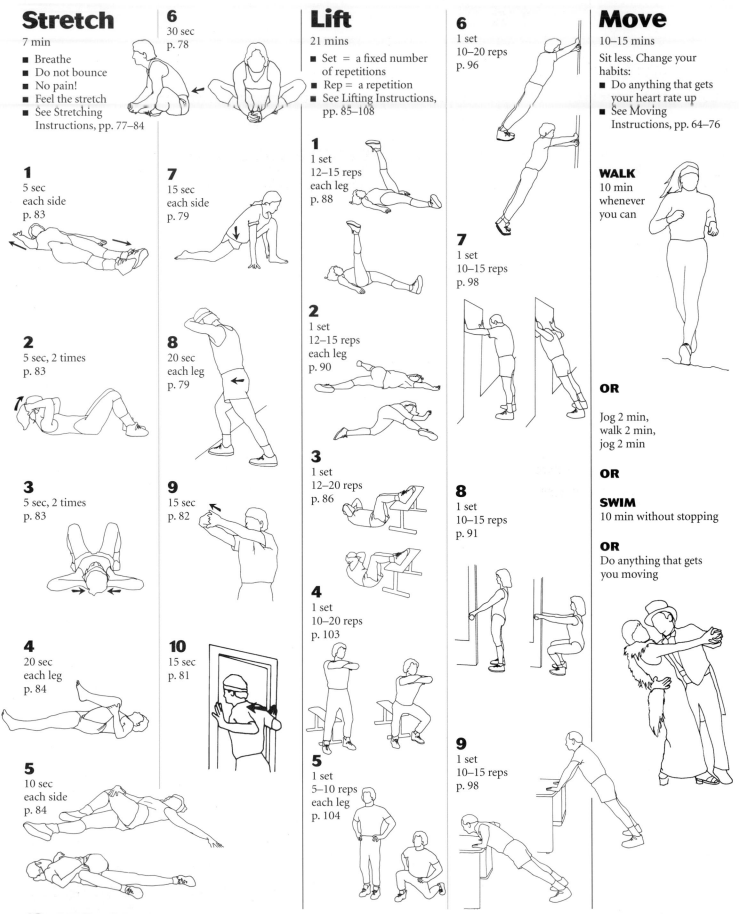

Stretch
7 min

- Breathe
- Do not bounce
- No pain!
- Feel the stretch
- See Stretching Instructions, pp. 77–84

1
5 sec
each side
p. 83

2
5 sec, 2 times
p. 83

3
5 sec, 2 times
p. 83

4
20 sec
each leg
p. 84

5
10 sec
each side
p. 84

6
30 sec
p. 78

7
15 sec
each side
p. 79

8
20 sec
each leg
p. 79

9
15 sec
p. 82

10
15 sec
p. 81

Lift
21 mins

- Set = a fixed number of repetitions
- Rep = a repetition
- See Lifting Instructions, pp. 85–108

1
1 set
12–15 reps
each leg
p. 88

2
1 set
12–15 reps
each leg
p. 90

3
1 set
12–20 reps
p. 86

4
1 set
10–20 reps
p. 103

5
1 set
5–10 reps
each leg
p. 104

6
1 set
10–20 reps
p. 96

7
1 set
10–15 reps
p. 98

8
1 set
10–15 reps
p. 91

9
1 set
10–15 reps
p. 98

Move
10–15 mins

Sit less. Change your habits:

- Do anything that gets your heart rate up
- See Moving Instructions, pp. 64–76

WALK
10 min
whenever
you can

OR

Jog 2 min,
walk 2 min,
jog 2 min

OR

SWIM
10 min without stopping

OR

Do anything that gets you moving

Photocopy this page and take it with you when you work out.

THE 5 BASIC PROGRAMS

THE HEART OF THIS BOOK

Turn the page and take a look at Basic Program 1. Start here if you feel you are in good enough shape or if you have already worked through the Program Before the Program.

HOW DO THE 5 BASIC PROGRAMS WORK?

- Each program is designed to prepare you for the next one.
- This gives you goals to shoot for.
- You'll have a clear path for steady progress.

WHEN DO I MOVE FROM ONE PROGRAM TO ANOTHER?

- Once you can do a program comfortably, go to the next level.
- *Rule of thumb:* Stick with each Basic Program for 4 to 6 weeks.

WHAT EQUIPMENT WILL I NEED?

Basic Program 1 requires only a barbell and two dumbbells, no bench. Basic Programs 2 to 5 have added a multi-purpose bench.

HOW MUCH DO I NEED TO DO?

We encourage you to follow these programs. They are carefully worked out and balanced. But feel free to substitute activities or skip any exercises that seem too difficult or cause pain. Also, you may want to advance to a certain level and go no further. That's okay, too. These are guidelines, not prescriptions. For example:

- You may want to do no more than stretch a few minutes a day.
- You may want to follow these graduated Basic Programs up to a certain point to achieve and maintain a certain level of fitness.
- Or, if you want to get really fit, you can work through Basic Program 5. By then you will be close to the American College of Sports Medicine's fitness guidelines for "healthy adults" *(see pp. 194–197).*

PACE YOURSELF

Your body is a remarkable organism and will surprise you with its ability to get stronger. But it can surprise you just as readily by breaking down if you overwork it. *Take it easy,* and as you progress through the 5 Basic Programs, your body will gradually adapt to the increasing levels of exercise. You will notice, and enjoy, the difference.

HERE'S BASIC PROGRAM 1 . . .

BASIC PROGRAM 1

Stretch

3 min

- Breathe
- Do not bounce
- No pain!
- *Feel* each stretch
- See Stretching Instructions, pp. 77–84

1
15 sec
p. 81

2
5 sec
2 times
p. 81

3
5 sec
each side
p. 84

4
5 sec
each side
p. 82

5
15 sec
each leg
p. 79

6
15 sec
each leg
p. 79

7
15 sec
each leg
p. 79

8
20 sec
p. 78

9
10 sec
each side
p. 78

10
15 sec
each leg
p. 84

11
5 sec
each side
p. 83

Move

15 min

- Don't get too far out of breath; you should be able to talk while exercising
- Remember the value of moderate exercise
- See Move Instructions, pp. 64–76

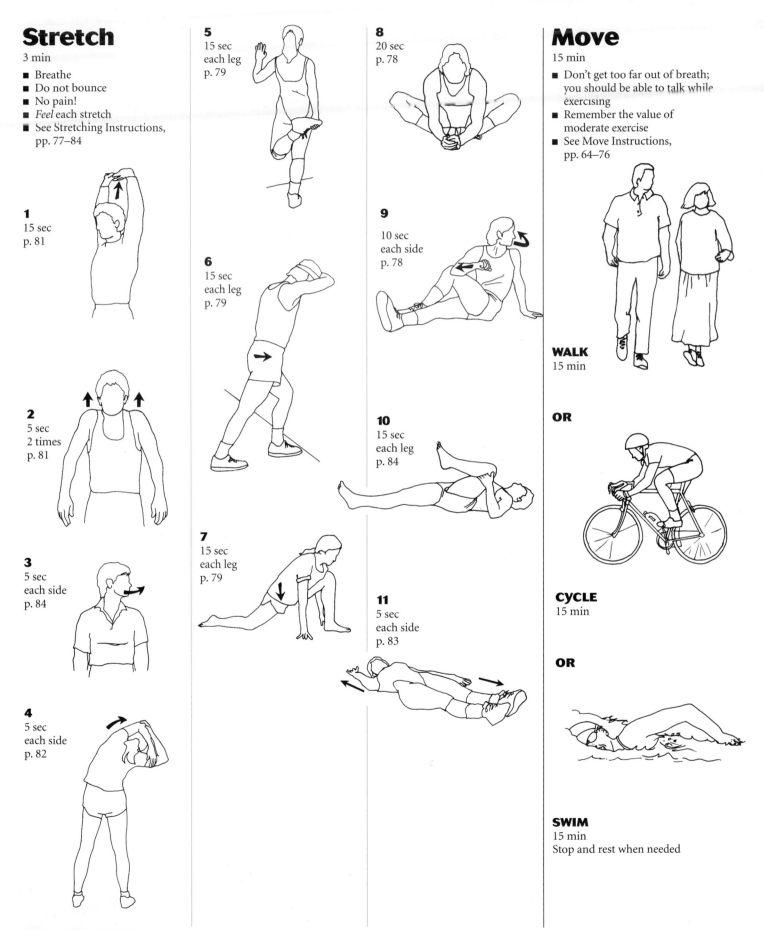

WALK
15 min

OR

CYCLE
15 min

OR

SWIM
15 min
Stop and rest when needed

Photocopy this page and take it with you when you work out.

BASIC PROGRAM 1

OR

Do anything
that gets you
moving.

Don't worry about heart rate.

ONE STEP AT A TIME

- Start by taking one extra
  step a day for a week.
- Continue to go a little
  farther than you did
  yesterday.
- You are the one who
  regulates the intensity of
  your progress.

TAKE IT EASY

Many people overdo physical
exercise and get bored or
hurt.

Too hard too soon may lead
to no exercise at all.

Lift

24 min

- Set = a fixed number of
  repetitions
- Rep = a repetition
- See Lifting Instructions,
  pp. 85–108

1
1 set
10–15 reps
p. 86

2
1 set
5–10 reps
each leg
p. 87

3
1 set
12 reps
p. 99

4
1 set
12 reps
p. 100

5
1 set
12 reps
p. 93

6
1 set
12 reps
p. 106

7
1 set
12 reps
p. 94

8
1 set
10–15 reps
p. 103

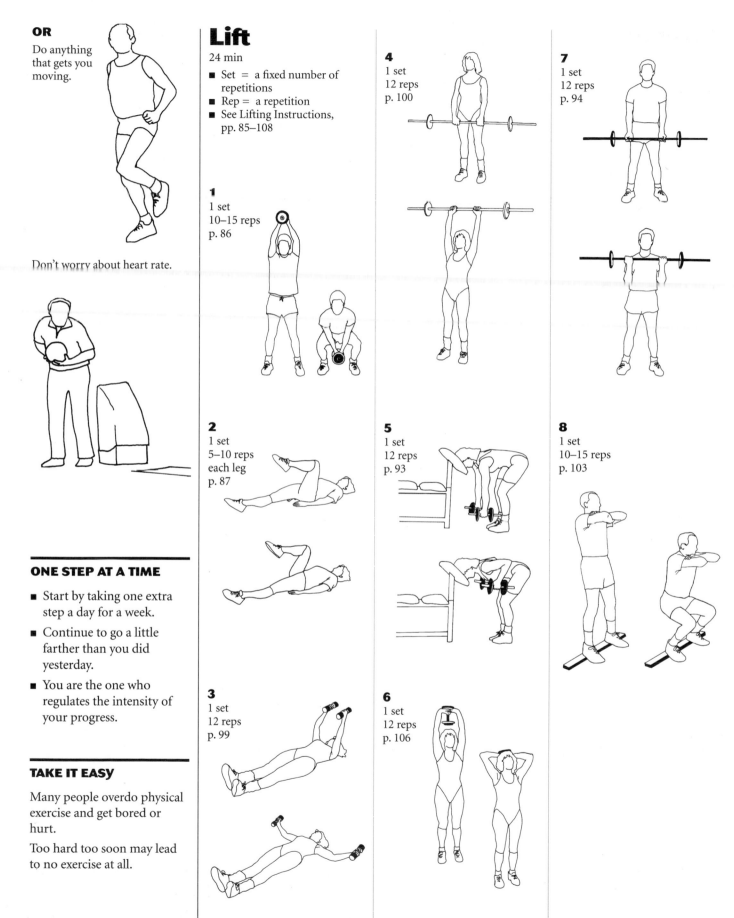

BASIC PROGRAM 2

Stretch and warm up first.
Cool down after.

Stretch

4 min
- Breathe
- Do not bounce
- No pain!
- Feel the stretch
- See Stretching Instructions, pp. 77–84

1
30 sec
p. 78

2
10 sec
p. 78

3
20 sec
each leg
p. 79

4
10 sec, 2 times
p. 81

5
5 sec, 2 times
p. 81

6
10 sec
each side
p. 82

7
10 sec
each side
p. 82

8
15 sec
each leg
p. 79

9
5–8 sec
p. 83

10
5 sec
each side
p. 83

Move

20–30 min
- Don't get too far out of breath; you should be able to talk while exercising
- Remember the value of moderate exercise
- See Move Instructions, pp. 64–76

WALK
25–30 min

**OR
CYCLE**
20–25 min

OR

SWIM
20–25 min
Stop and rest when needed.

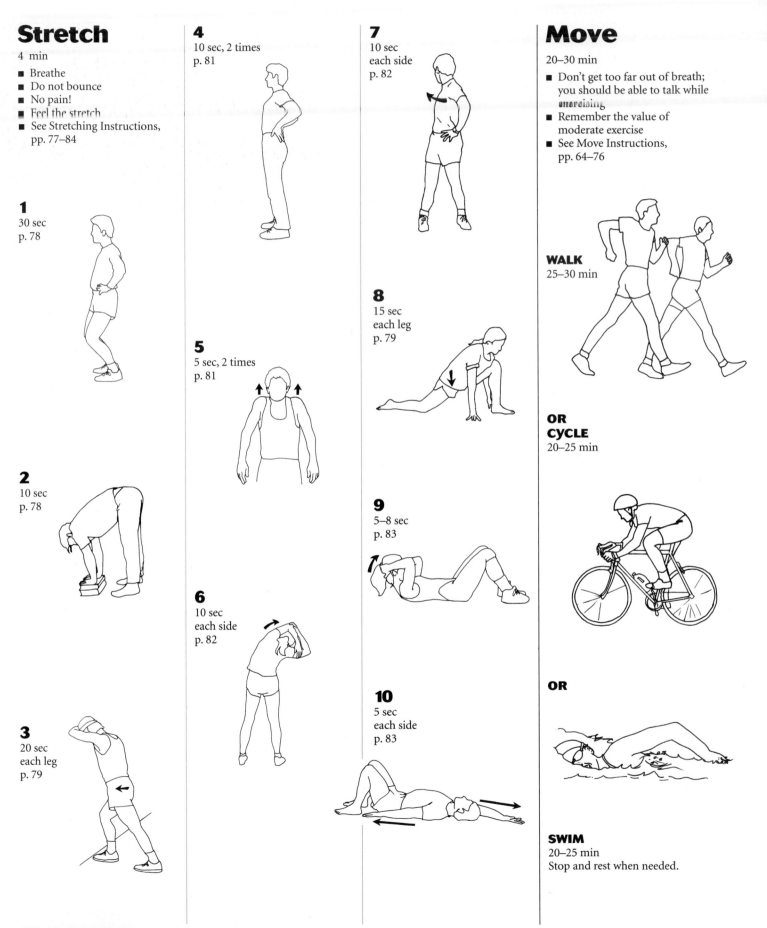

Photocopy this page and take it with you when you work out.

BASIC PROGRAM 2

OR

Move for 20–30 min at least 2–3 times a week.

Working is a workout: gardening, housecleaning, building, washing the car, shoveling snow.

- Lawn mowing is a good way to burn calories.
- Gardening uses almost as many calories as moderate swimming.

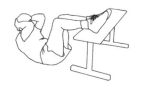

FITNESS IS AN ONGOING PROCESS

- It's a direction.
- Don't be rigid.
- You're on your way.

TAKE IT EASY

Slow, steady progression will result in improved fitness.

Lift
26 min

- Set = a fixed number of repetitions
- Rep = a repetition
- Use enough weight so last rep of set is slightly difficult
- Increase weights only when last rep is not strenuous
- Never lift to failure
- See Lifting Instructions, pp. 85–108

1
1 set 10–20 reps
each side
p. 86

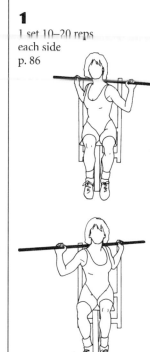

2
1 set
5–15 reps
p. 86

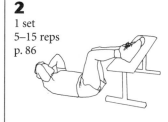

3
1 set
12 reps
p. 103

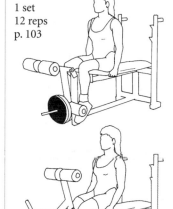

4
1 set
12 reps
p. 99

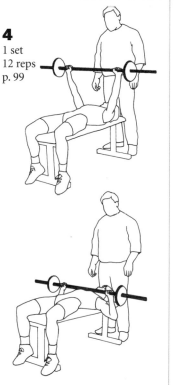

5
1 set
12 reps
p. 100

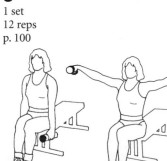

6
1 set
12 reps
p. 93

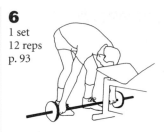

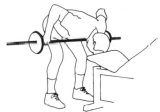

7
1 set
12 reps
p. 106

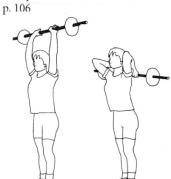

8
1 set
12 reps
p. 95

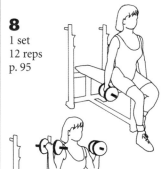
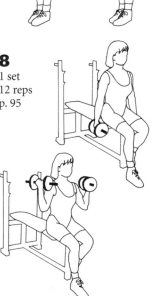

BASIC PROGRAM 3

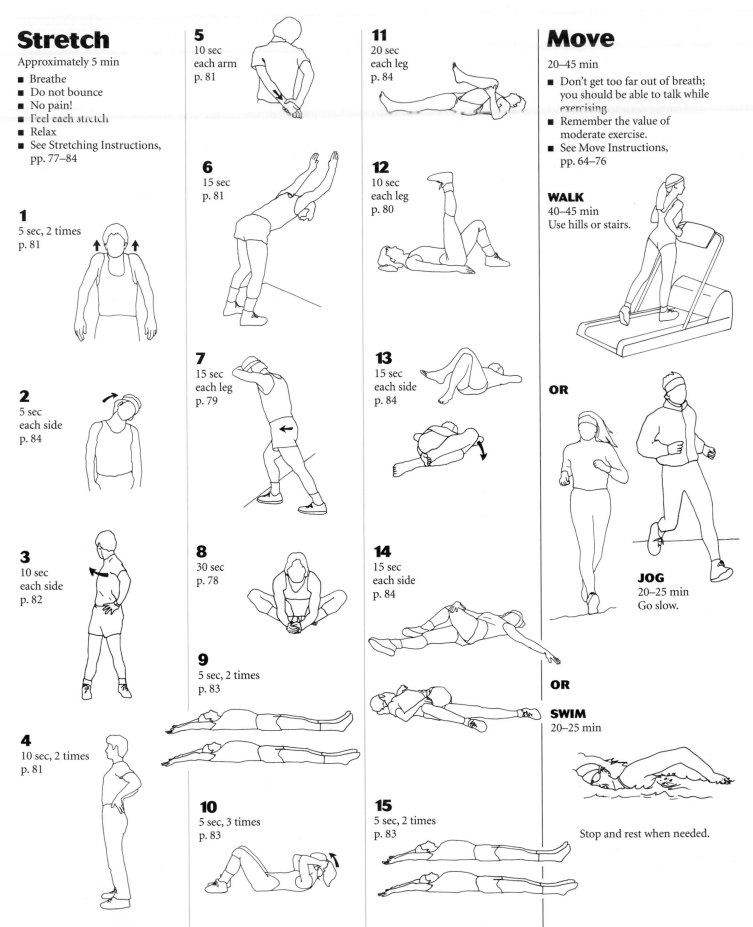

Stretch

Approximately 5 min

- Breathe
- Do not bounce
- No pain!
- Feel each stretch
- Relax
- See Stretching Instructions, pp. 77–84

1
5 sec, 2 times
p. 81

2
5 sec
each side
p. 84

3
10 sec
each side
p. 82

4
10 sec, 2 times
p. 81

5
10 sec
each arm
p. 81

6
15 sec
p. 81

7
15 sec
each leg
p. 79

8
30 sec
p. 78

9
5 sec, 2 times
p. 83

10
5 sec, 3 times
p. 83

11
20 sec
each leg
p. 84

12
10 sec
each leg
p. 80

13
15 sec
each side
p. 84

14
15 sec
each side
p. 84

15
5 sec, 2 times
p. 83

Move

20–45 min

- Don't get too far out of breath; you should be able to talk while exercising
- Remember the value of moderate exercise.
- See Move Instructions, pp. 64–76

WALK
40–45 min
Use hills or stairs.

OR

JOG
20–25 min
Go slow.

OR

SWIM
20–25 min

Stop and rest when needed.

Photocopy this page and take it with you when you work out.

Stretch every day.
Lift OR Move on alternate days.

BASIC PROGRAM 3

OR

Mix activities: walk one day, garden another day, etc.

How you move is not as important as *that* you move.

Think of anything you want to do or have to do where you can move.

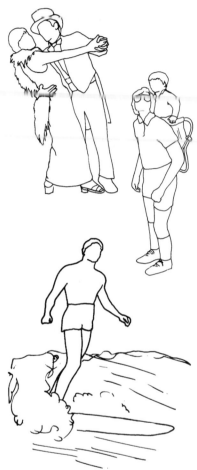

THE SPICE OF LIFE

- Do different things. Exercise in different ways.
- For both mind and body, change your routine every 4–6 weeks.
- If something you are doing becomes stale, stop doing it. Switch to another activity.

Just get your heart rate up

Lift

28 min

- Set = a fixed number of repetitions
- Rep = a repetition
- Use enough weight so last rep of set is slightly difficult
- Increase weights only when last rep is not strenuous
- Never lift to failure
- See Lifting Instructions, pp. 85–108

1
1 set
15–30 reps
p. 86

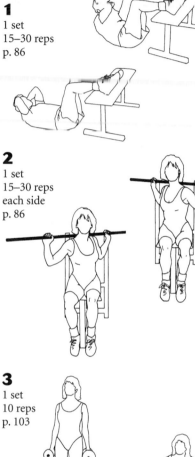

2
1 set
15–30 reps
each side
p. 86

3
1 set
10 reps
p. 103

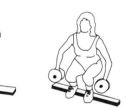

4
1 set
10 reps
p. 97

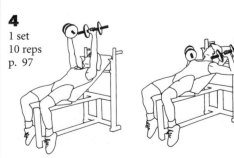

5
1 set
10 reps
p. 97

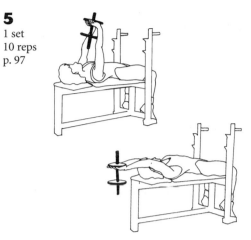

6
1 set
10 reps
p. 100

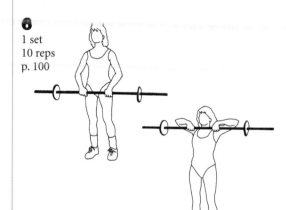

7
1 set
10 reps
p. 107

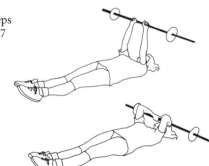

8
1 set
10 reps
each arm
p. 94

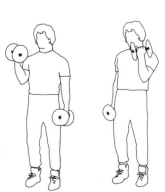

BASIC PROGRAM 4

**Stretch and warm up first.
Cool down after.**

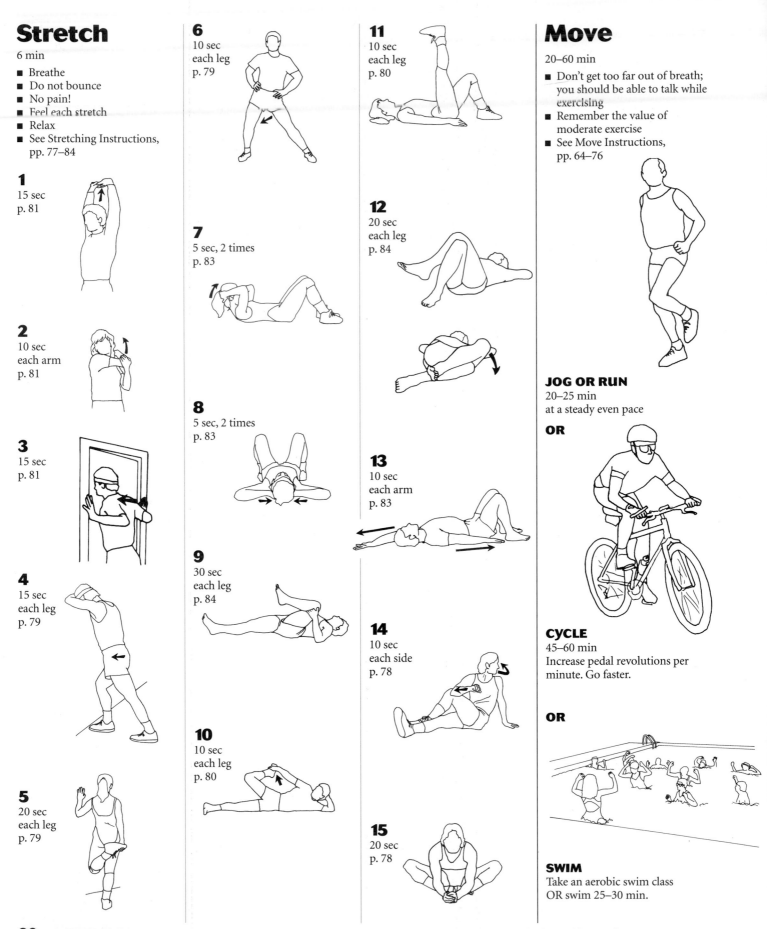

Stretch

6 min

- Breathe
- Do not bounce
- No pain!
- Feel each stretch
- Relax
- See Stretching Instructions, pp. 77–84

1
15 sec
p. 81

2
10 sec
each arm
p. 81

3
15 sec
p. 81

4
15 sec
each leg
p. 79

5
20 sec
each leg
p. 79

6
10 sec
each leg
p. 79

7
5 sec, 2 times
p. 83

8
5 sec, 2 times
p. 83

9
30 sec
each leg
p. 84

10
10 sec
each leg
p. 80

11
10 sec
each leg
p. 80

12
20 sec
each leg
p. 84

13
10 sec
each arm
p. 83

14
10 sec
each side
p. 78

15
20 sec
p. 78

Move

20–60 min

- Don't get too far out of breath; you should be able to talk while exercising
- Remember the value of moderate exercise
- See Move Instructions, pp. 64–76

JOG OR RUN
20–25 min
at a steady even pace

OR

CYCLE
45–60 min
Increase pedal revolutions per minute. Go faster.

OR

SWIM
Take an aerobic swim class
OR swim 25–30 min.

Photocopy this page and take it with you when you work out.

Stretch every day.
Lift OR Move on alternate days.

OR

Do aerobics: Stair–stepping, Lifecycle, treadmill, aerobic dance.

Go roller skating or bowling.

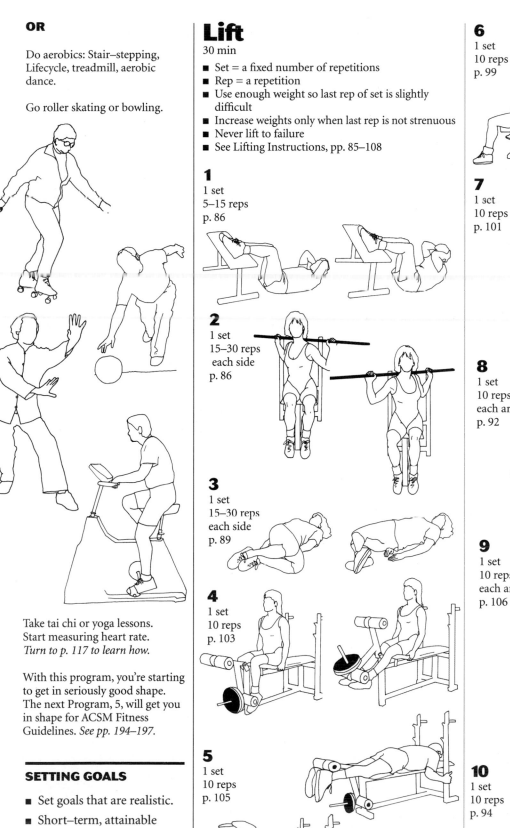

Take tai chi or yoga lessons. Start measuring heart rate. *Turn to p. 117 to learn how.*

With this program, you're starting to get in seriously good shape. The next Program, 5, will get you in shape for ACSM Fitness Guidelines. *See pp. 194–197.*

SETTING GOALS

- Set goals that are realistic.
- Short–term, attainable goals can get you through the day.
- Long–term, ambitious goals can give you hope for the future.

Lift

30 min

- Set = a fixed number of repetitions
- Rep = a repetition
- Use enough weight so last rep of set is slightly difficult
- Increase weights only when last rep is not strenuous
- Never lift to failure
- See Lifting Instructions, pp. 85–108

1
1 set
5–15 reps
p. 86

2
1 set
15–30 reps
each side
p. 86

3
1 set
15–30 reps
each side
p. 89

4
1 set
10 reps
p. 103

5
1 set
10 reps
p. 105

6
1 set
10 reps
p. 99

7
1 set
10 reps
p. 101

8
1 set
10 reps
each arm
p. 92

9
1 set
10 reps
each arm
p. 106

10
1 set
10 reps
p. 94

Photocopy this page and take it with you when you work out.

BASIC PROGRAM 5

**Stretch and warm up first.
Cool down after.**

Stretch
7 min

- Breathe
- No bouncing or forcing
- No pain
- Pay attention to how each stretch feels
- Relax
- See Stretching Instructions, pp. 77–84

1
5 sec, 2 times
each side
p. 83

2
5 sec, 2 times
p. 83

3
5 sec, 2 times
p. 83

4
25 sec
each leg
p. 84

5
15 sec
each side
p. 82

6
10 sec, 2 times
p. 82

7
15 sec
each leg
p. 78

8
10 sec
each leg
p. 80

9
15 sec
each leg
p. 80

10
20 sec
each leg
p. 79

11
30 sec
p. 78

12
15 sec
p. 78

13
10 sec
p. 81

14
15 sec
p. 82

15
10 sec
each side
p. 82

16
20 sec
each leg
p. 79

17
10 sec
p. 81

Move
30–60 min

- Don't get too far out of breath; you should be able to talk while exercising
- Remember the value of moderate exercise
- See Move Instructions, pp. 64–76

RUN
30 min or more

OR

CYCLE
60 min or more
Increase pedal revolutions to 70–90 per min

OR

SWIM
25 min or longer — fast, without stopping to rest.

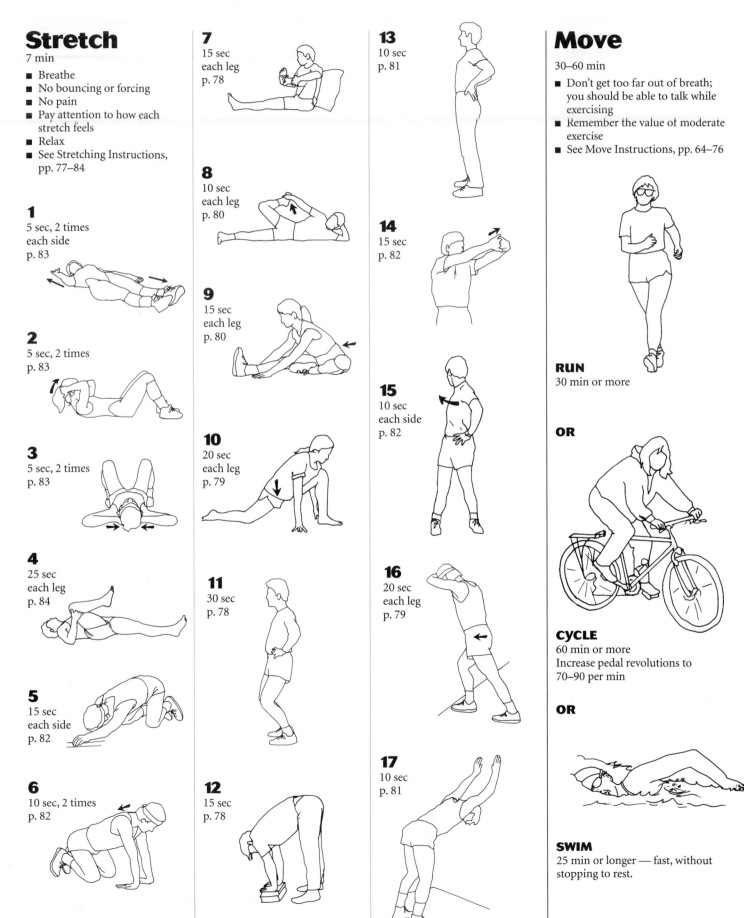

Photocopy this page and take it with you when you work out.

BASIC PROGRAM 5

OR

Play sports: tennis, basketball, ice skating, soccer, skiing, surfing. Or do some useful labor.

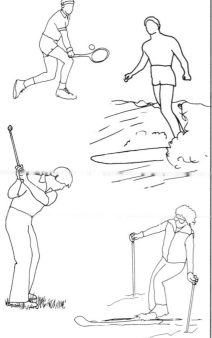

Continue measuring heart rate. *See p. 117 to learn how.* Once you can do this program, you are up to the ACSM Fitness Guidelines. *See pp. 194–197.*

ACTIVATE ENDORPHINS

The best-known exercise-induced brain change is the release of *endorphins,* chemical substances 20 times more powerful than morphine, from the pituitary gland. Vigorous workouts can increase endorphins by as much as 5 times.

A CURE FOR DEPRESSION

Physical activity doesn't cure depression, says Dr. Robert Brown of the University of Virginia, but lack of exercise causes it. In fact, confinement and physical inactivity are traditional punishments.

Lift

38 min

- Set = a fixed number of repetitions
- Rep = a repetition
- Use enough weight so last rep of set is slightly difficult
- Increase weights only when last rep is easy
- Never lift to failure
- See Lifting Instructions, pp. 85–108

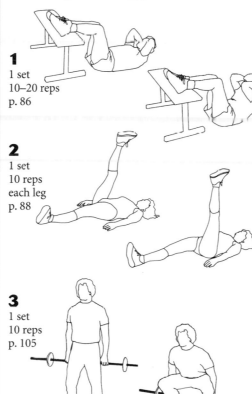

1
1 set
10–20 reps
p. 86

2
1 set
10 reps
each leg
p. 88

3
1 set
10 reps
p. 105

4
1 set
10 reps
p. 105

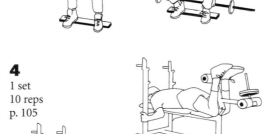

5
1 set
10 reps
p. 99

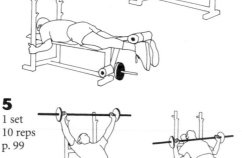

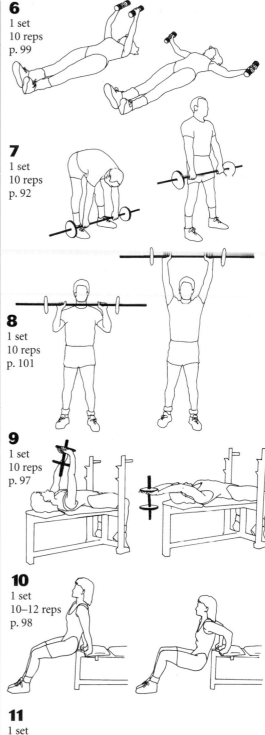

6
1 set
10 reps
p. 99

7
1 set
10 reps
p. 92

8
1 set
10 reps
p. 101

9
1 set
10 reps
p. 97

10
1 set
10–12 reps
p. 98

11
1 set
10 reps
p. 95

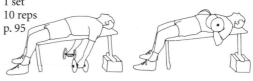

12
1 set
10 reps
p. 86

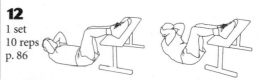

Energy spent mowing the lawn counts as much as that used on a three-mile run. And the exertion you use playing a fun game of softball or volleyball with the guys after work is just as good as that spent on the rowing machine — even if your heart doesn't pound the whole time. Spent the weekend cleaning the house? It counts. So does digging in the garden, raking leaves, grocery shopping, walking the dog, playing badminton with the kids, fixing the car or dancing.

Even activity on the job — moving stock, fixing pipes, climbing utility poles, chasing after 3-year olds — counts.

Porter Shimer
co-author of *Fitness Without Exercise,*
as reported in the *Los Angeles Times*

SPECIAL PROGRAMS

Note: *You should be at Level 3 of the Program Before the Program (p. 18) before you try any of these Programs. For Circuit Training, it's advisable to be at the level of Basic Program 2 (pp. 22–23).*

Basic Programs 1–5 are the foundation for a sound and graduated approach to getting (back) in shape. However, there are certain situations or goals that call for special programs.

ON THE JOB AND DESK STRETCHES

Programs that can be done on a break at work. Primarily for people with desk jobs *(pp. 33–35)*.

THE BUSY DAY

For those days when you can't fit in a 30–40 min workout at one time. You take 2 to 3 very short (10–15 min) workouts *(pp. 36–37)*.

ON THE ROAD

For travelers. Stretches to do on the plane, exercises to do in a hotel room, at the airport, in the car, or anywhere away from home *(pp. 38–40)*.

STRETCH & STRENGTHEN

Three unique programs consisting of a stretch, then an exercise, another stretch, another exercise, and so on. These are the first such programs ever shown in a book *(pp. 41–44)*.

CIRCUIT TRAINING

Two weight training programs designed to give you an *aerobic* workout with weights. In circuit training, you do not rest between exercises. You move rapidly through the carefully sequenced exercises to keep your heart rate up *(pp. 45–47)*.

ELECTRONIC GYM

Two programs using the LifeCircuit system of weight training. One uses free weights in combination with LifeCircuit *(pp. 48–51)*.

HEALTH CONDITIONS

Programs designed to ease back pain *(p. 151)* and arthritis *(p. 147)* and one for weight management *(p. 178)*.

THE VALUE OF MODERATE EXERCISE

The image and standard of vigorous, sweat-soaked exercise has discouraged many sedentary individuals from even trying to become more active. The bulk of benefit may come from expending as little as 500 calories a week in moderate physical exercise. And such activity need not be an arduous bout of exercise, but can be pleasurable, enjoyable activities: talking, gardening, bowling, dancing, golf, and so on.

—Dr. David Sobel
Healthy People 2000

ON THE JOB

There are lots of things you can do to burn extra calories on the job, reduce the discomfort of some workplaces, and make yourself feel better during the work day.

Exercise at work will benefit employers as well as employees — in reduced absenteeism and health-care costs. Productivity tends to increase when employees stretch or exercise at work. Studies have shown that small amounts of moderate exercise lead to increased energy and decreased tension for several hours after activity.

STRETCHING This is the easiest activity to do at work.

LIFTING How to strengthen and tone your muscles at work? Carry a briefcase or purse in your hand rather than using a shoulder strap. Do a biceps curl with a heavy book. Do some isometric exercises while sitting in a chair. Be creative.

MOVING

- *Mini-walks.* Take a longer route to the bathroom or photocopier. Walk during coffee breaks. Walk to talk to a colleague instead of using the phone.

- *Climb more stairs.* Take the stairs instead of the elevator. You burn 4 calories for every 10 steps you climb.

- *Park and walk.* Park a distance away from work instead of as close as you can get. Walking burns calories. Or when you go shopping, park on the outskirts of the mall parking lot. Give up the car ride to the station in the morning and walk to the bus or train.

- *Stand and talk.* While talking on the phone, stand up and pace for a few minutes. Pacing burns about one calorie for every 15–20 steps you take. Stretch to ease upper body tension.

- *Wear comfortable shoes.* The latest well-designed walking shoes feel so great you'll be encouraged to walk farther and more often. Choose a quality, light pair of dress walking shoes to wear at work. Or, keep a pair of running or walking shoes at the office to use during lunch hour walks.

- *Elevate feet each day for 3–5 minutes.* Good for circulation and relief for swollen, tired feet. Also helps prevent varicose veins.

DESK STRETCHES

These are stretches to do at your desk.
This program will take 2 1/2 – 3 min.

- Breathe easily
- No bouncing or forcing
- No pain!
- *Feel* the stretch
- Relax
- See Stretching Instructions, pp. 77–84

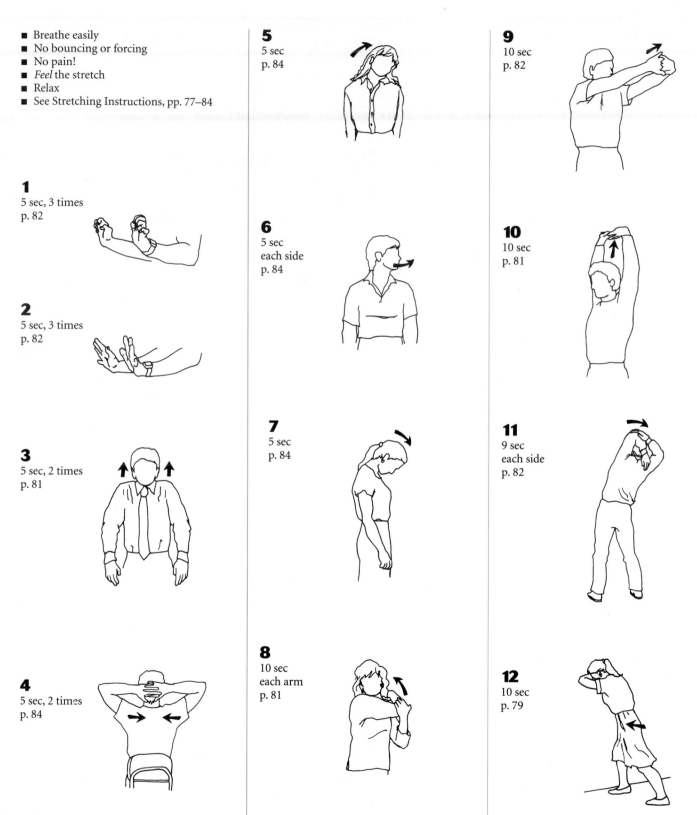

1
5 sec, 3 times
p. 82

2
5 sec, 3 times
p. 82

3
5 sec, 2 times
p. 81

4
5 sec, 2 times
p. 84

5
5 sec
p. 84

6
5 sec
each side
p. 84

7
5 sec
p. 84

8
10 sec
each arm
p. 81

9
10 sec
p. 82

10
10 sec
p. 81

11
9 sec
each side
p. 82

12
10 sec
p. 79

- Prolonged sitting at a desk or computer terminal can cause muscular tension and pain.
- Taking a few minutes to do a series of stretches can make your whole body feel better.
- Learn to stretch spontaneously throughout the day whenever you feel tense.
- Don't just do seated stretches, but do some standing stretches too. Good for circulation.

Photocopy this page and keep it in your desk drawer.

This program is for people who either sit or stand every day at work.
This program will take 5–15 min.

ON THE JOB

Stretch

3 min

- Always stretch and warm up before you exercise
- Do not bounce
- No pain!
- *Feel* each stretch
- See Stretching Instructions, pp. 77–84

1
15 sec
p. 81

2
10 sec
p. 82

3
15 sec
each leg
p. 79

4
15 sec
each leg
p. 79

5
15 sec
p. 81

6
5 sec, 3 times
p. 82

7
5 sec, 2 times
p. 81

8
15 sec
p. 81

9
5 sec
each side
p. 84

10
10 sec
p. 79

Lift

12 min

- Set = a fixed number of repetitions
- Rep = a repetition
- See Lifting Instructions, pp. 85–108

1
1 set
10–20 reps
p. 105

2
1 set
15–20 reps
p. 98

3
1 set
8–12 reps
p. 91

4
1 set
2–12 reps
p. 98

5
1 set
10–25 reps
p. 87

Move

10–20 min

- Do anything that gets your heart rate up
- See Moving Instructions, pp. 64–76

RUN IN PLACE
10 min

OR

WALK DURING LUNCH
20 min

OR

WALK WITH WEIGHTS
15 min

OR

CLIMB STAIRS
3 times a day

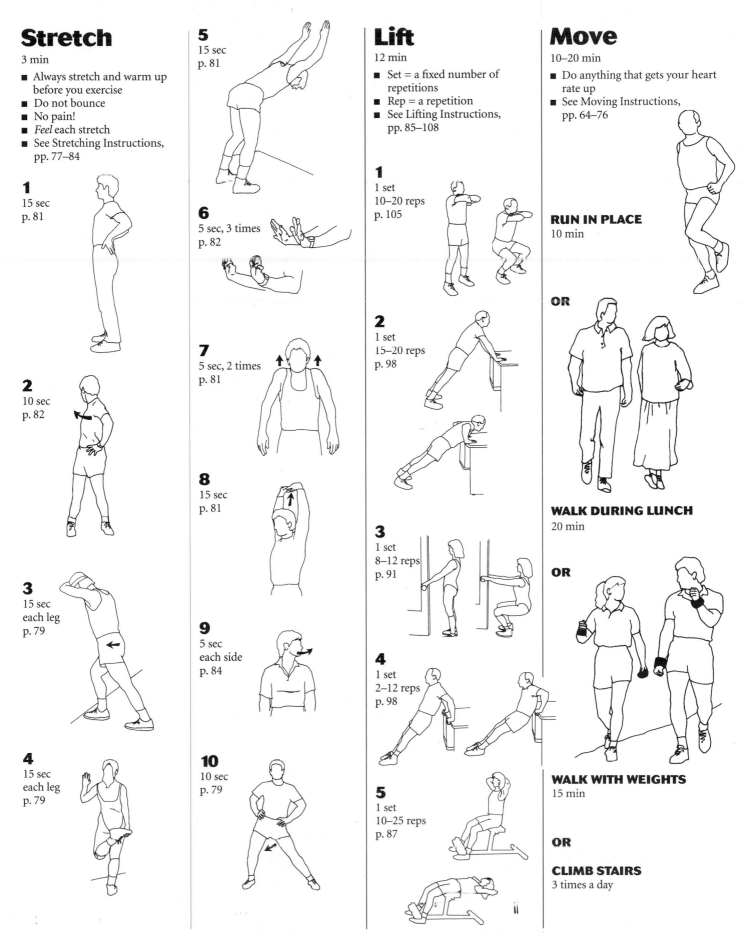

Photocopy this page and keep it at your workplace

THE BUSY DAY

Although light to moderate physical activity for a sustained period of at least 30 minutes is preferable, intermittent physical activity also increases caloric expenditure and may be important for those who cannot fit 30 minutes of sustained activity into their schedules.

Healthy People 2000
U.S. Dept. of Health and Human Services

TAKE 10

Can't even get in a 30-minute workout some days? Well, take three 10-minute workouts instead. Recent research has shown that three 10-minute workouts provide almost as much health benefit as one 30-minute workout.

> *When you don't have enough time for a full workout, several short sessions are better than none at all.*

YOU WON'T LOSE GROUND

Think of these sessions as *maintenance:* three short 10-minute sessions will keep you in shape until you can get back to your regular program.

MAKE A FITNESS APPOINTMENT

Busy, successful executives often find ways to include exercise in their already crowded life-styles. Schedule exercise for a time when an interruption is least likely. An in-house gym certainly helps. Make — and keep — an appointment with exercise every day, just like your other business appointments.

MIX AND MATCH

- Walk for 2–10 minutes three times a day
- Mix strength exercises, stair climbing and stretching
- Ride a stationary bike 5–10–15 minutes at a time
- Stretch when watching the news

Avoid scheduled, intense exercise routines and instead substitute small bouts of activity spaced comfortably throughout the day.

THE BUSY DAY

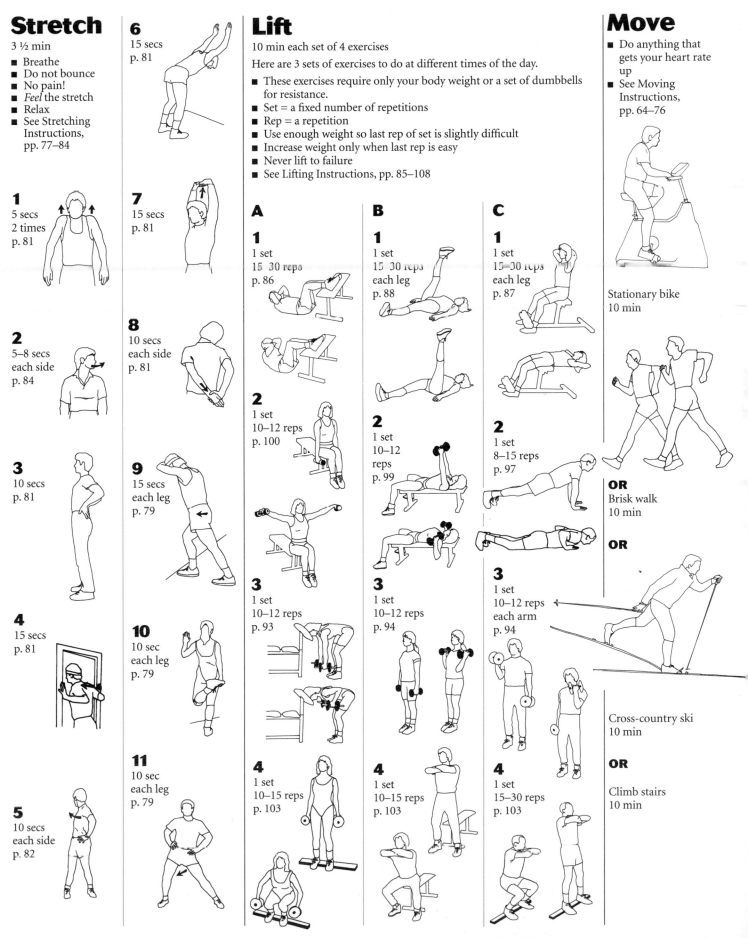

Stretch

3 ½ min

- Breathe
- Do not bounce
- No pain!
- *Feel* the stretch
- Relax
- See Stretching Instructions, pp. 77–84

1
5 secs
2 times
p. 81

2
5–8 secs
each side
p. 84

3
10 secs
p. 81

4
15 secs
p. 81

5
10 secs
each side
p. 82

6
15 secs
p. 81

7
15 secs
p. 81

8
10 secs
each side
p. 81

9
15 secs
each leg
p. 79

10
10 sec
each leg
p. 79

11
10 sec
each leg
p. 79

Lift

10 min each set of 4 exercises

Here are 3 sets of exercises to do at different times of the day.

- These exercises require only your body weight or a set of dumbbells for resistance.
- Set = a fixed number of repetitions
- Rep = a repetition
- Use enough weight so last rep of set is slightly difficult
- Increase weight only when last rep is easy
- Never lift to failure
- See Lifting Instructions, pp. 85–108

A

1
1 set
15–30 reps
p. 86

2
1 set
10–12 reps
p. 100

3
1 set
10–12 reps
p. 93

4
1 set
10–15 reps
p. 103

B

1
1 set
15–30 reps
each leg
p. 88

2
1 set
10–12 reps
p. 99

3
1 set
10–12 reps
p. 94

4
1 set
10–15 reps
p. 103

C

1
1 set
15–30 reps
each leg
p. 87

2
1 set
8–15 reps
p. 97

3
1 set
10–12 reps
each arm
p. 94

4
1 set
15–30 reps
p. 103

Move

- Do anything that gets your heart rate up
- See Moving Instructions, pp. 64–76

Stationary bike
10 min

OR

Brisk walk
10 min

OR

Cross-country ski
10 min

OR

Climb stairs
10 min

Photocopy this page and keep it in your desk drawer.

ON THE ROAD

In the plane, on a long car ride, or in the hotel room, you stiffen up from sitting for long periods of time. During long flights, you get dehydrated. It's worse when flights are three hours or longer, when the normal rhythms of your daily activities are disrupted.

ON THE PLANE

- *Move around* and stretch to relieve sore muscles.
- *Drink lots of fluid.* Coffee + alcohol = dehydration. Drink mineral water, juices, soda.
- *Eat lightly.* You'll feel better and adjust more quickly. Eat fruit and vegetables, not heavy and/or salty foods. Bring a turkey sandwich.
- *Airport exercise:* Walk to your flight instead of taking the airport shuttle. Stretch while waiting around. Some airports have in-house gyms. You can often squeeze in a workout between flights.

DURING CAR TRIPS

Every few hours, get out and walk a bit. Stretch. Once again, eat light meals. Get to your room in time to exercise before your first appointment.

IN THE HOTEL ROOM

Pack an elastic exercise band and a jump rope with your luggage and start the morning before business with a few minutes of jumping and strength exercises.

Many hotels now have gyms. (Check on this when making reservations.) However if there is no gym, the program on p. 40 will provide a quick hotel room workout.

ENERGY IN THE ACT

You'll find energy in the workout itself. When you get off the plane and get to your hotel, you think, "Oh, I'm so tired." But just push yourself out that door. Tune in to your new environment. It doesn't have to be an hour run. It can be a 15-minute walk. Get moving. You'll feel better. It will do a lot for jet lag and make you more alert for the business you came to conduct.

ON THE ROAD: AIRPLANE STRETCHES

Stretch

Approximately 3½ min

- Breathe
- Do not bounce
- No pain!
- *Feel* the stretch
- Relax
- See Stretching Instructions, pp. 77–84

1
10 sec
2 times
p. 82

2
5 sec
p. 81

3
10 sec
p. 81

4
5 sec
each side
p. 84

5
5 sec
each side
p. 84

6
10 sec
each arm
p. 81

7
10 sec
p. 82

8
15 sec
each leg
p. 79

9
10 sec
each leg
p. 79

10
10 sec
each leg
p. 79

11
10 times
each direction
each foot
p. 79

12
10 sec
each side
p. 82

13
10 sec
p. 81

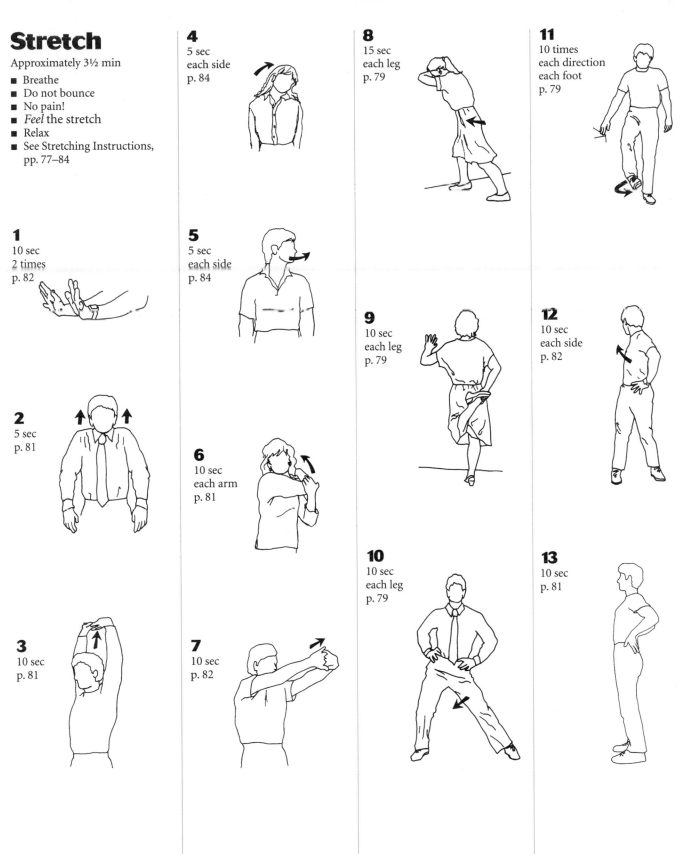

Photocopy this page and take it on the airplane with you.

ON THE ROAD: HOTEL ROOM WORKOUT

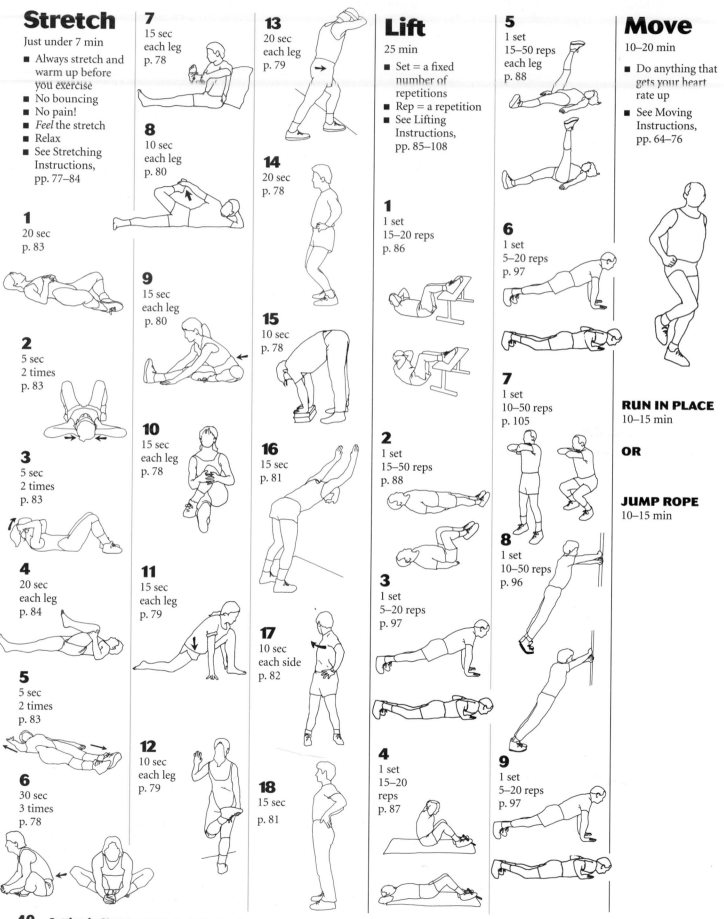

Stretch

Just under 7 min

- Always stretch and warm up before you exercise
- No bouncing
- No pain!
- *Feel* the stretch
- Relax
- See Stretching Instructions, pp. 77–84

1
20 sec
p. 83

2
5 sec
2 times
p. 83

3
5 sec
2 times
p. 83

4
20 sec
each leg
p. 84

5
5 sec
2 times
p. 83

6
30 sec
3 times
p. 78

7
15 sec
each leg
p. 78

8
10 sec
each leg
p. 80

9
15 sec
each leg
p. 80

10
15 sec
each leg
p. 78

11
15 sec
each leg
p. 79

12
10 sec
each leg
p. 79

13
20 sec
each leg
p. 79

14
20 sec
p. 78

15
10 sec
p. 78

16
15 sec
p. 81

17
10 sec
each side
p. 82

18
15 sec
p. 81

Lift

25 min

- Set = a fixed number of repetitions
- Rep = a repetition
- See Lifting Instructions, pp. 85–108

1
1 set
15–20 reps
p. 86

2
1 set
15–50 reps
p. 88

3
1 set
5–20 reps
p. 97

4
1 set
15–20 reps
p. 87

5
1 set
15–50 reps
each leg
p. 88

6
1 set
5–20 reps
p. 97

7
1 set
10–50 reps
p. 105

8
1 set
10–50 reps
p. 96

9
1 set
5–20 reps
p. 97

Move

10–20 min

- Do anything that gets your heart rate up
- See Moving Instructions, pp. 64–76

RUN IN PLACE
10–15 min

OR

JUMP ROPE
10–15 min

Photocopy this page and take it with you when you travel.

STRETCH & STRENGTHEN

These are three unique programs. In fact, there is no other book that shows stretching interspersed with weight training exercises.

- Here, the emphasis is on flexibility along with a weight training workout. You do a stretch, then an exercise. While you're resting from the exercise you do another stretch, and so on.

- Even if you don't do a stretch & strengthen workout, there's often time in between sets to stretch (for example, in a busy gym, or when training with a partner). Stretch while you're waiting to do the next exercise. Stretch the same muscles you're exercising. Be creative.

- *After a while, you can make up your own stretch & strengthen programs.* It's simple: take any of the programs in the book and do the stretches indicated between the exercises, rather than all together.

STRETCH & STRENGTHEN 1

Stretch & Lift

Stretch time: 3 min
Lift time: 25 min

- Stretch, then do the lifting exercise
- While you are resting from the lift, do the next stretch
- And so on, until you complete all 9 combinations in this program
- When you feel strong enough, move on to Stretch & Strengthen 2

STRETCHING

- Always stretch and warm up before you exercise
- Do not bounce
- No pain
- See Stretching Instructions, pp. 77–84

LIFTING

- Set = a fixed number of repetitions
- Rep = a repetition
- Use enough weight so last rep of set is slightly difficult
- Increase weight only when last rep is not strenuous
- Never lift to failure
- See Lifting Instructions, pp. 85–108

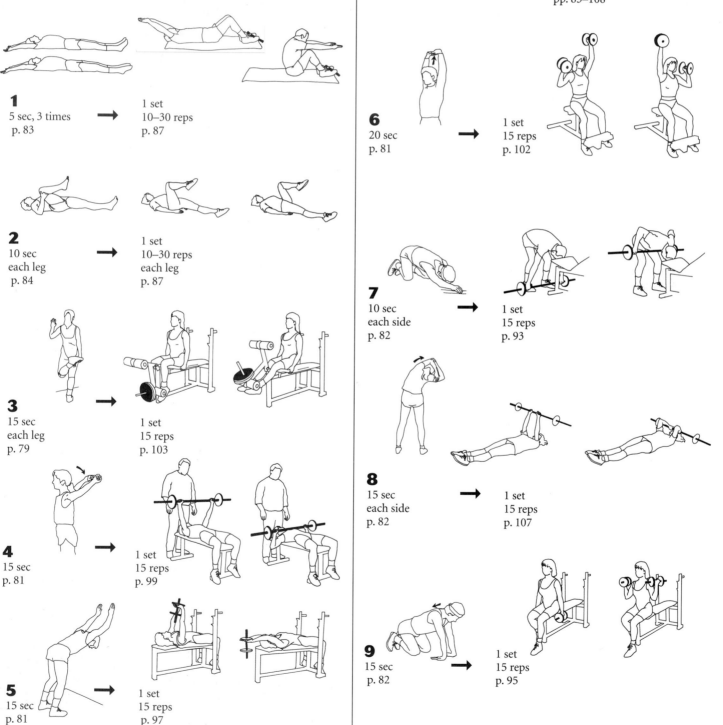

1
5 sec, 3 times
p. 83
→ 1 set
10–30 reps
p. 87

2
10 sec
each leg
p. 84
→ 1 set
10–30 reps
each leg
p. 87

3
15 sec
each leg
p. 79
→ 1 set
15 reps
p. 103

4
15 sec
p. 81
→ 1 set
15 reps
p. 99

5
15 sec
p. 81
→ 1 set
15 reps
p. 97

6
20 sec
p. 81
→ 1 set
15 reps
p. 102

7
10 sec
each side
p. 82
→ 1 set
15 reps
p. 93

8
15 sec
each side
p. 82
→ 1 set
15 reps
p. 107

9
15 sec
p. 82
→ 1 set
15 reps
p. 95

STRETCH & STRENGTHEN 2

Stretch & Lift

Stretch time: 4 min
Lift time: 30 min

- Stretch, then do the lifting exercise
- While you are resting from the lift, do the next stretch
- And so on, until you complete all 11 combinations in this program
- When you feel strong enough, move on to Stretch & Strengthen 3

STRETCHING

- Always stretch and warm up before you exercise
- Do not bounce
- No pain!
- See Stretching Instructions, pp. 77–84

LIFTING

- Set = a fixed number of repetitions
- Rep = a repetition
- Use enough weight so last rep of set is slightly difficult.
- Increase weight only when last rep is not strenuous.
- Never lift to failure.
- See Lifting Instructions, pp. 85–108

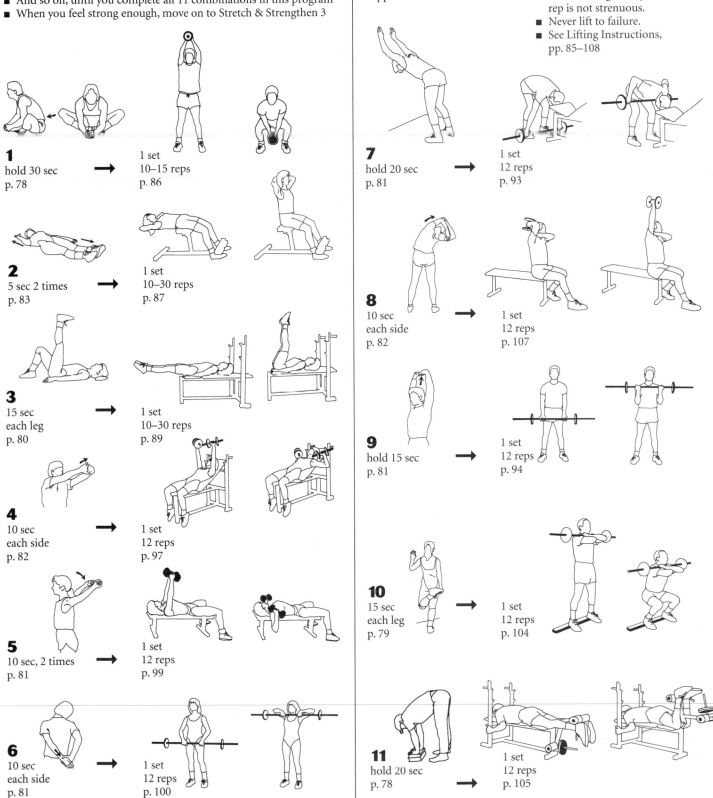

1
hold 30 sec
p. 78
→
1 set
10–15 reps
p. 86

2
5 sec 2 times
p. 83
→
1 set
10–30 reps
p. 87

3
15 sec
each leg
p. 80
→
1 set
10–30 reps
p. 89

4
10 sec
each side
p. 82
→
1 set
12 reps
p. 97

5
10 sec, 2 times
p. 81
→
1 set
12 reps
p. 99

6
10 sec
each side
p. 81
→
1 set
12 reps
p. 100

7
hold 20 sec
p. 81
→
1 set
12 reps
p. 93

8
10 sec
each side
p. 82
→
1 set
12 reps
p. 107

9
hold 15 sec
p. 81
→
1 set
12 reps
p. 94

10
15 sec
each leg
p. 79
→
1 set
12 reps
p. 104

11
hold 20 sec
p. 78
→
1 set
12 reps
p. 105

Photocopy this page and take it with you when you work out.

STRETCH & STRENGTHEN 3

Stretch & Lift

Stretch time: 5 min
Lift time: 40 min

- Stretch, then do the lifting exercise
- While you are resting from the lift, do the next stretch
- And so on, until you complete all 14 combinations in this program

STRETCHING

- Always stretch and warm up before you exercise
- Do not bounce
- No pain!
- See Stretching Instructions, pp. 77–84

LIFTING

- Set = a fixed number of repetitions
- Rep = a repetition
- Use enough weight so last rep of set is slightly difficult
- Increase weight only when last rep is not strenuous
- Never lift to failure
- See Lifting Instructions, pp. 85–108

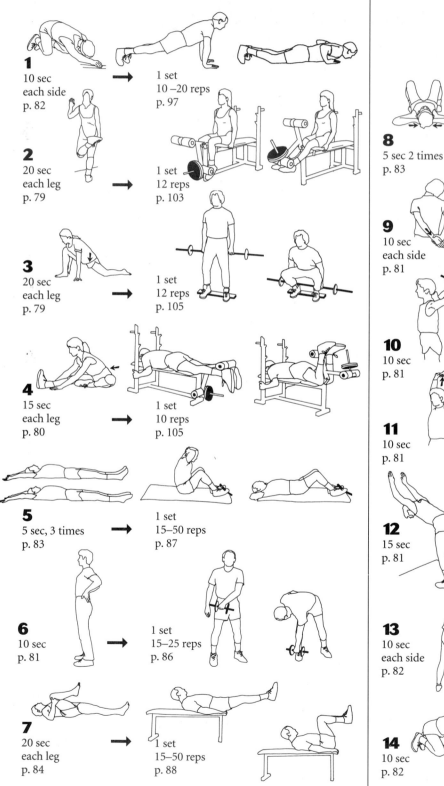

1
10 sec each side
p. 82
→ 1 set
10–20 reps
p. 97

2
20 sec each leg
p. 79
→ 1 set
12 reps
p. 103

3
20 sec each leg
p. 79
→ 1 set
12 reps
p. 105

4
15 sec each leg
p. 80
→ 1 set
10 reps
p. 105

5
5 sec, 3 times
p. 83
→ 1 set
15–50 reps
p. 87

6
10 sec
p. 81
→ 1 set
15–25 reps
p. 86

7
20 sec each leg
p. 84
→ 1 set
15–50 reps
p. 88

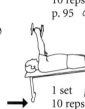
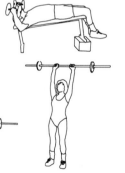
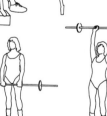
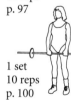
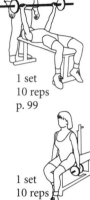
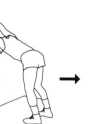
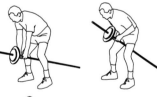
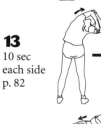
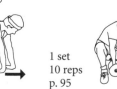

8
5 sec 2 times
p. 83
→ 1 set
10 reps
p. 99

9
10 sec each side
p. 81
→ 1 set
10 reps
p. 95

10
10 sec
p. 81
→ 1 set
10 reps
p. 97

11
10 sec
p. 81
→ 1 set
10 reps
p. 100

12
15 sec
p. 81
→ 1 set
10 reps
p. 93

13
10 sec each side
p. 82
→ 1 set
10 reps
p. 107

14
10 sec
p. 82
→ 1 set
10 reps
p. 95

Photocopy this page and take it with you when you work out.

CIRCUIT TRAINING

Circuit training means using weight training to get an aerobic workout.

In general, weight training programs develop:
- Muscular endurance
- Muscular strength

Circuit training develops:
- Muscular endurance
- Muscular strength
- Cardiovascular endurance

HOW DOES IT WORK?

- You move quickly from one exercise to the next.
- Equipment is set up so you can move from one exercise to the next quickly. You either use a multi-station machine or set up free weights so you can do one exercise right after the other.
- You monitor your pulse so your heart rate stays at 50% of maximum target heart rate or higher during the entire workout (*see pp. 116–118*).

CHECK WITH YOUR DOCTOR

These are strenuous programs, so be sure to get your doctor's approval first.

STRETCH FIRST

Always stretch before training.

BASIC CIRCUIT TRAINING

In these programs, do 3–6 min of aerobic conditioning before starting the programs to bring your heart rate to target zone level. After doing exercise 1, immediately do exercise 2, and so on. With as little rest as necessary, do all the exercises. The idea is to get your heart rate up and keep it there.

SUPER CIRCUIT TRAINING

In this program, you do *supersets:* one exercise quickly followed by 30 sec to 2 min on a stationary bike, treadmill, or stair climber.

BASIC CIRCUIT TRAINING

This program will take 30–35 min.

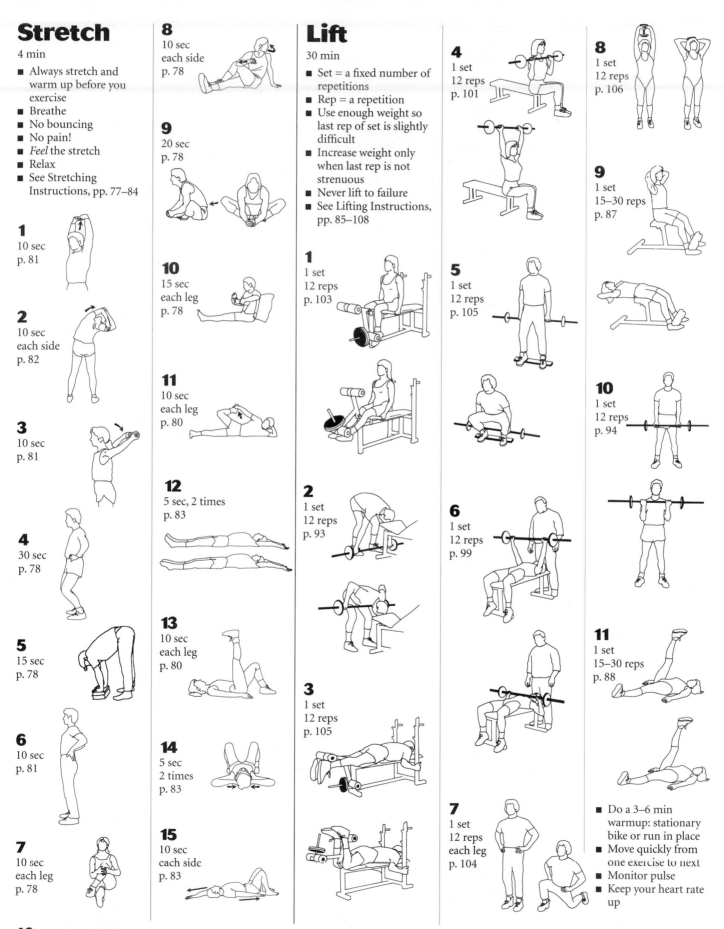

Stretch

4 min

- Always stretch and warm up before you exercise
- Breathe
- No bouncing
- No pain!
- *Feel* the stretch
- Relax
- See Stretching Instructions, pp. 77–84

1
10 sec
p. 81

2
10 sec
each side
p. 82

3
10 sec
p. 81

4
30 sec
p. 78

5
15 sec
p. 78

6
10 sec
p. 81

7
10 sec
each leg
p. 78

8
10 sec
each side
p. 78

9
20 sec
p. 78

10
15 sec
each leg
p. 78

11
10 sec
each leg
p. 80

12
5 sec, 2 times
p. 83

13
10 sec
each leg
p. 80

14
5 sec
2 times
p. 83

15
10 sec
each side
p. 83

Lift

30 min

- Set = a fixed number of repetitions
- Rep = a repetition
- Use enough weight so last rep of set is slightly difficult
- Increase weight only when last rep is not strenuous
- Never lift to failure
- See Lifting Instructions, pp. 85–108

1
1 set
12 reps
p. 103

2
1 set
12 reps
p. 93

3
1 set
12 reps
p. 105

4
1 set
12 reps
p. 101

5
1 set
12 reps
p. 105

6
1 set
12 reps
p. 99

7
1 set
12 reps
each leg
p. 104

8
1 set
12 reps
p. 106

9
1 set
15–30 reps
p. 87

10
1 set
12 reps
p. 94

11
1 set
15–30 reps
p. 88

- Do a 3–6 min warmup: stationary bike or run in place
- Move quickly from one exercise to next
- Monitor pulse
- Keep your heart rate up

Getting in Shape © 1994 Shelter Publications, Inc.

Photocopy this page and take it with you when you work out.

SUPER CIRCUIT TRAINING

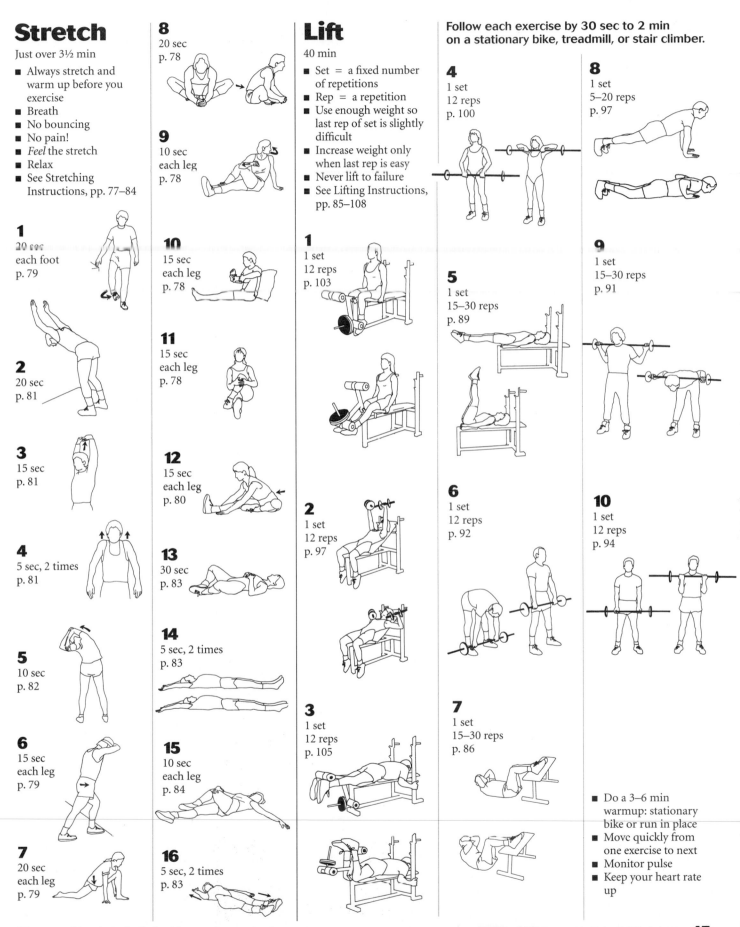

Stretch

Just over 3½ min

- Always stretch and warm up before you exercise
- Breath
- No bouncing
- No pain!
- *Feel* the stretch
- Relax
- See Stretching Instructions, pp. 77–84

1
20 sec
each foot
p. 79

2
20 sec
p. 81

3
15 sec
p. 81

4
5 sec, 2 times
p. 81

5
10 sec
p. 82

6
15 sec
each leg
p. 79

7
20 sec
each leg
p. 79

8
20 sec
p. 78

9
10 sec
each leg
p. 78

10
15 sec
each leg
p. 78

11
15 sec
each leg
p. 78

12
15 sec
each leg
p. 80

13
30 sec
p. 83

14
5 sec, 2 times
p. 83

15
10 sec
each leg
p. 84

16
5 sec, 2 times
p. 83

Lift

40 min

- Set = a fixed number of repetitions
- Rep = a repetition
- Use enough weight so last rep of set is slightly difficult
- Increase weight only when last rep is easy
- Never lift to failure
- See Lifting Instructions, pp. 85–108

1
1 set
12 reps
p. 103

2
1 set
12 reps
p. 97

3
1 set
12 reps
p. 105

Follow each exercise by 30 sec to 2 min on a stationary bike, treadmill, or stair climber.

4
1 set
12 reps
p. 100

5
1 set
15–30 reps
p. 89

6
1 set
12 reps
p. 92

7
1 set
15–30 reps
p. 86

8
1 set
5–20 reps
p. 97

9
1 set
15–30 reps
p. 91

10
1 set
12 reps
p. 94

- Do a 3–6 min warmup: stationary bike or run in place
- Move quickly from one exercise to next
- Monitor pulse
- Keep your heart rate up

Photocopy this page and take it with you when you work out.

THE ELECTRONIC GYM

A revolutionary type of weight training machine has appeared in the past few years. These machines are markedly different from anything in the past and offer advantages hitherto unavailable. First, let's look briefly at the evolution of strength training equipment in America:

- The '50s: free weights
- The '60s: Universal-type machines (weight stacks and cables)
- The '70s: Nautilus-type machines (variable resistance cams)
- The '90s: Computerized resistance machines

LIFECIRCUIT MACHINES

Life Fitness, the company that makes the popular LifeCycle (a computerized exercycle) has recently come out with a line of 12 electronic workout machines called the LifeCircuit. These machines are unique in the field so we'll describe how they operate and how they're different.

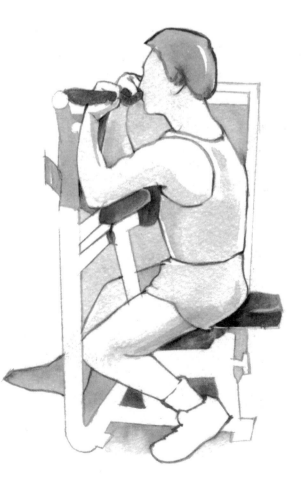

TWO BASIC PRINCIPLES
OF ELECTRONIC WORKOUT MACHINES

The two basic things that differ are:

- There is a computerized console that you program.
- Resistance is electromagnetic; that is, the amount of weight you lift is determined by varying amounts of electronic resistance.

The built-in computer controls electronic resistance tailored to your individual needs. In this way, the machine acts like a personal trainer.

HERE'S HOW THEY WORK

You sit down at the machine and take a simple strength test. The computer records your current strength in its memory and sets up a program tailored to give you maximum benefit. As you do the exercises, lights on the console change color as you complete each rep correctly. LED windows show the level of resistance converted into pounds.

ADVANTAGES

- Workout time is minimal. You can actually work eight major muscle groups in as little as 15 minutes.
- There are no plates to move, pins to insert and there is less risk of injury from falling weights or incorrect weight selection.
- The machines provide *negative* resistance: you not only *lift* the weight *up*, you must *resist* the weight as it moves *down*.
- You can choose between a regular program and a "pyramid" program that is more difficult.
- Workouts are fun. The machines are bringing new people into the gyms. Kids, brought up on video games, love the machines, and older people appreciate the low-impact workout.

The machines are expensive — some $70,000 for the full set, so you obviously won't have them at home, and only the larger gyms will have them. But if you can locate a gym that carries them, go in for a test and see for yourself what the electronic age has done for weight training.

LIFECIRCUIT TRAINING

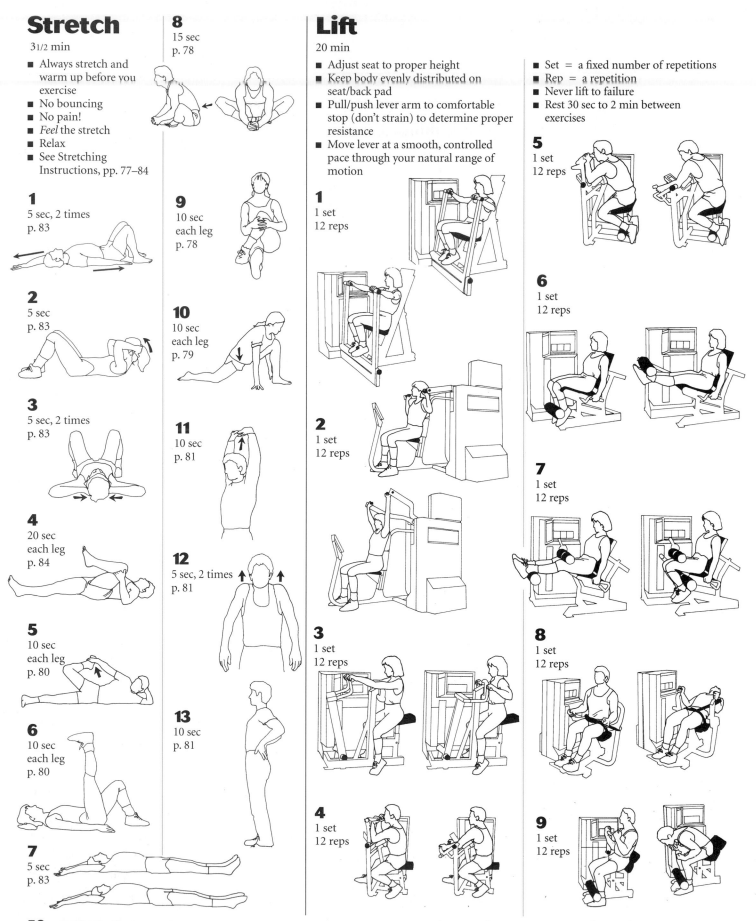

Stretch

3 1/2 min

- Always stretch and warm up before you exercise
- No bouncing
- No pain!
- *Feel* the stretch
- Relax
- See Stretching Instructions, pp. 77–84

1
5 sec, 2 times
p. 83

2
5 sec
p. 83

3
5 sec, 2 times
p. 83

4
20 sec
each leg
p. 84

5
10 sec
each leg
p. 80

6
10 sec
each leg
p. 80

7
5 sec
p. 83

8
15 sec
p. 78

9
10 sec
each leg
p. 78

10
10 sec
each leg
p. 79

11
10 sec
p. 81

12
5 sec, 2 times
p. 81

13
10 sec
p. 81

Lift

20 min

- Adjust seat to proper height
- Keep body evenly distributed on seat/back pad
- Pull/push lever arm to comfortable stop (don't strain) to determine proper resistance
- Move lever at a smooth, controlled pace through your natural range of motion

- Set = a fixed number of repetitions
- Rep = a repetition
- Never lift to failure
- Rest 30 sec to 2 min between exercises

1
1 set
12 reps

2
1 set
12 reps

3
1 set
12 reps

4
1 set
12 reps

5
1 set
12 reps

6
1 set
12 reps

7
1 set
12 reps

8
1 set
12 reps

9
1 set
12 reps

Photocopy this page and take it with you when you work out.

LIFECIRCUIT + FREE WEIGHTS

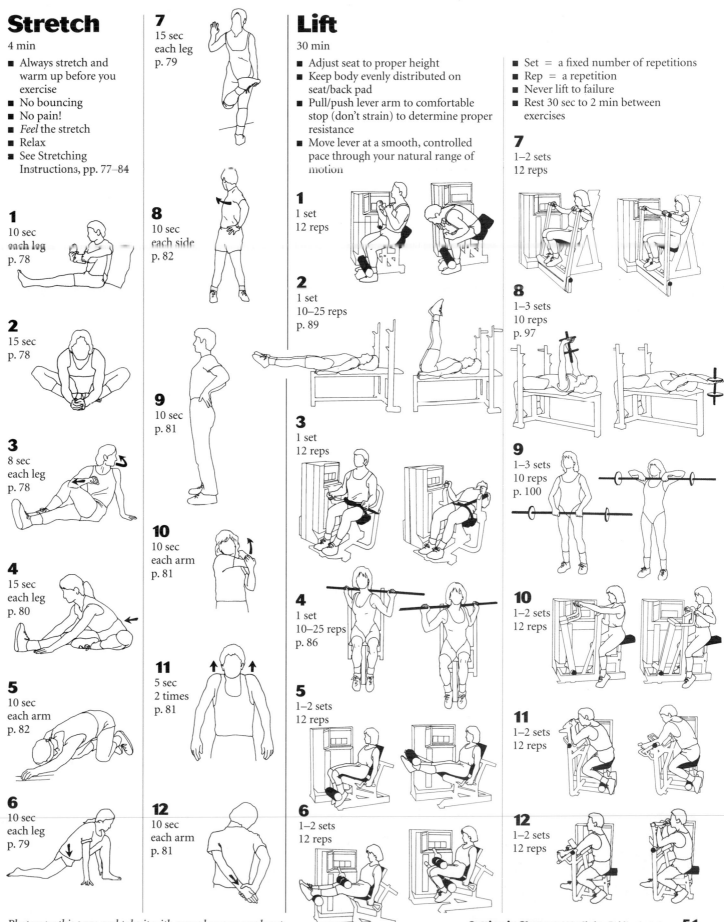

Stretch

4 min

- Always stretch and warm up before you exercise
- No bouncing
- No pain!
- *Feel* the stretch
- Relax
- See Stretching Instructions, pp. 77–84

1
10 sec each leg
p. 78

2
15 sec
p. 78

3
8 sec each leg
p. 78

4
15 sec each leg
p. 80

5
10 sec each arm
p. 82

6
10 sec each leg
p. 79

7
15 sec each leg
p. 79

8
10 sec each side
p. 82

9
10 sec
p. 81

10
10 sec each arm
p. 81

11
5 sec 2 times
p. 81

12
10 sec each arm
p. 81

Lift

30 min

- Adjust seat to proper height
- Keep body evenly distributed on seat/back pad
- Pull/push lever arm to comfortable stop (don't strain) to determine proper resistance
- Move lever at a smooth, controlled pace through your natural range of motion

- Set = a fixed number of repetitions
- Rep = a repetition
- Never lift to failure
- Rest 30 sec to 2 min between exercises

1
1 set
12 reps

2
1 set
10–25 reps
p. 89

3
1 set
12 reps

4
1 set
10–25 reps
p. 86

5
1–2 sets
12 reps

6
1–2 sets
12 reps

7
1–2 sets
12 reps

8
1–3 sets
10 reps
p. 97

9
1–3 sets
10 reps
p. 100

10
1–2 sets
12 reps

11
1–2 sets
12 reps

12
1–2 sets
12 reps

Photocopy this page and take it with you when you work out.

Getting in Shape © 1994 Shelter Publications, Inc. **51**

TESTS FOR WELLNESS

These six tests should be performed regularly:

- **Hearing** = every 2 years
- **Blood pressure** = every 2–5 years
- **Cholesterol** = every 5 years after age 18, more often for middle-aged men
- **Mammogram** = every 1–2 years between 40 – 49, annually after age 50
- **Eye exam** = every 2–5 years after age 40
- **Pap smear** = annually for women over 18 or who are sexually active

FINE TUNING

The following eight programs emphasize individual muscle groups. These are *overall body programs*, with exercises for all major muscle groups and emphasis on one body part. If you want to concentrate on muscular arms, for example, follow the Arms programs; if you want tighter buttocks, follow the Buttocks program, and so on.

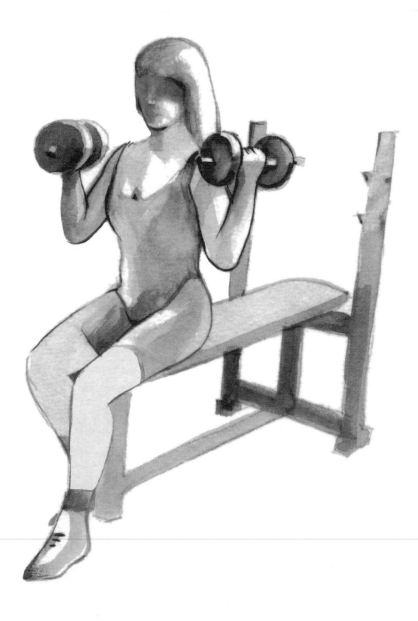

FINE TUNING: ABDOMINALS

This is a program of stretches and weight lifting exercises for overall body flexibility and strength, with special emphasis on the midsection.

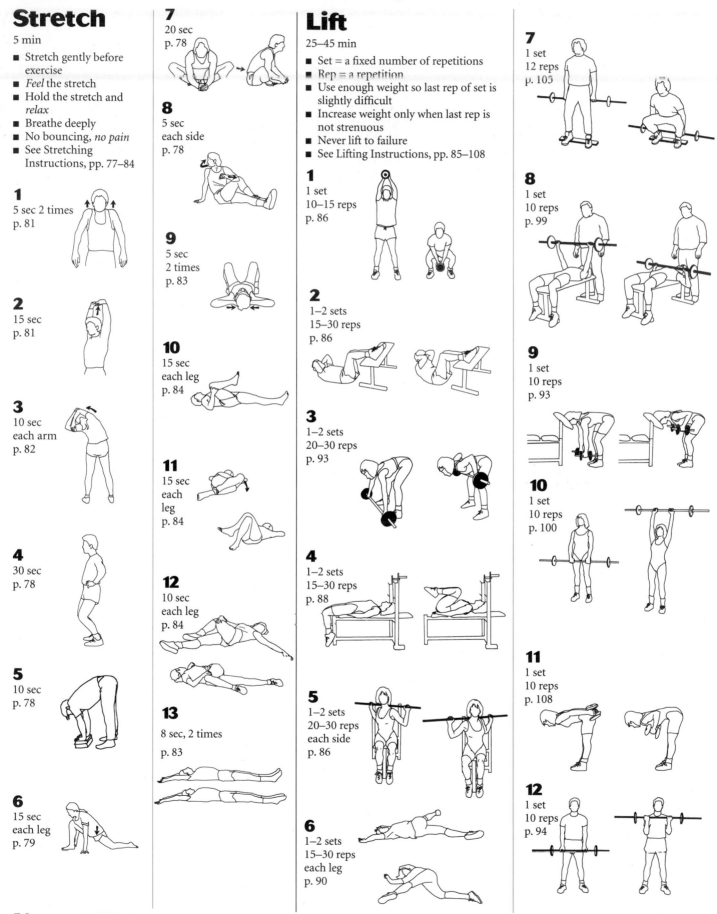

Stretch

5 min

- Stretch gently before exercise
- *Feel* the stretch
- Hold the stretch and *relax*
- Breathe deeply
- No bouncing, *no pain*
- See Stretching Instructions, pp. 77–84

1
5 sec 2 times
p. 81

2
15 sec
p. 81

3
10 sec
each arm
p. 82

4
30 sec
p. 78

5
10 sec
p. 78

6
15 sec
each leg
p. 79

7
20 sec
p. 78

8
5 sec
each side
p. 78

9
5 sec
2 times
p. 83

10
15 sec
each leg
p. 84

11
15 sec
each leg
p. 84

12
10 sec
each leg
p. 84

13
8 sec, 2 times
p. 83

Lift

25–45 min

- Set = a fixed number of repetitions
- Rep = a repetition
- Use enough weight so last rep of set is slightly difficult
- Increase weight only when last rep is not strenuous
- Never lift to failure
- See Lifting Instructions, pp. 85–108

1
1 set
10–15 reps
p. 86

2
1–2 sets
15–30 reps
p. 86

3
1–2 sets
20–30 reps
p. 93

4
1–2 sets
15–30 reps
p. 88

5
1–2 sets
20–30 reps
each side
p. 86

6
1–2 sets
15–30 reps
each leg
p. 90

7
1 set
12 reps
p. 105

8
1 set
10 reps
p. 99

9
1 set
10 reps
p. 93

10
1 set
10 reps
p. 100

11
1 set
10 reps
p. 108

12
1 set
10 reps
p. 94

 © 1994 Shelter Publications, Inc.   *Photocopy this page and take it with you when you work out.*

FINE TUNING: ARMS

This is a program of stretches and weight lifting exercises for overall body flexibility and strength, with special emphasis on the arms.

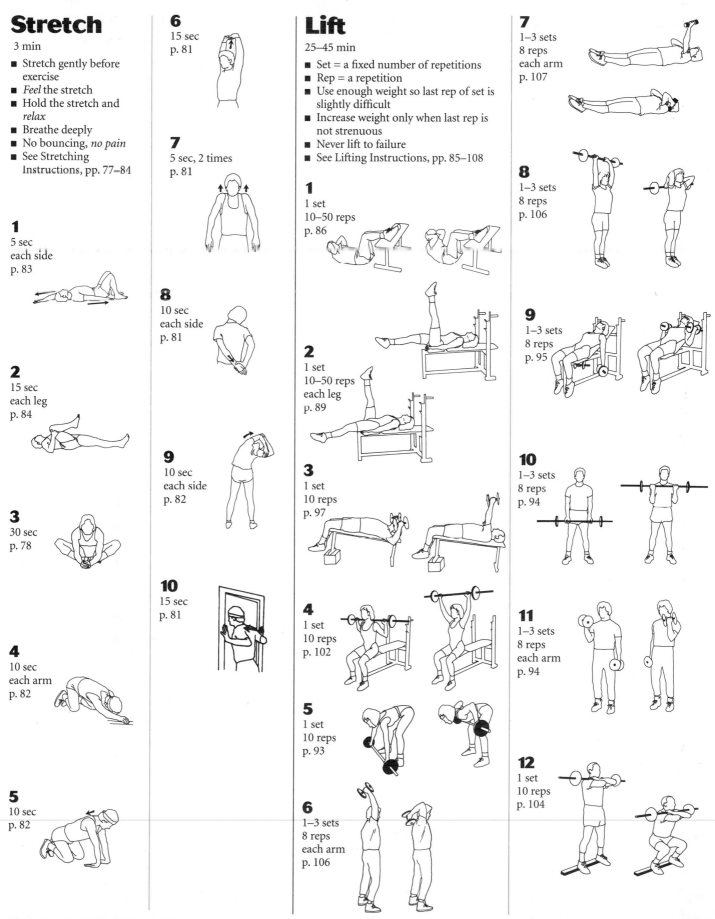

Stretch

3 min

- Stretch gently before exercise
- *Feel* the stretch
- Hold the stretch and *relax*
- Breathe deeply
- No bouncing, *no pain*
- See Stretching Instructions, pp. 77–84

1
5 sec
each side
p. 83

2
15 sec
each leg
p. 84

3
30 sec
p. 78

4
10 sec
each arm
p. 82

5
10 sec
p. 82

6
15 sec
p. 81

7
5 sec, 2 times
p. 81

8
10 sec
each side
p. 81

9
10 sec
each side
p. 82

10
15 sec
p. 81

Lift

25–45 min

- Set = a fixed number of repetitions
- Rep = a repetition
- Use enough weight so last rep of set is slightly difficult
- Increase weight only when last rep is not strenuous
- Never lift to failure
- See Lifting Instructions, pp. 85–108

1
1 set
10–50 reps
p. 86

2
1 set
10–50 reps
each leg
p. 89

3
1 set
10 reps
p. 97

4
1 set
10 reps
p. 102

5
1 set
10 reps
p. 93

6
1–3 sets
8 reps
each arm
p. 106

7
1–3 sets
8 reps
each arm
p. 107

8
1–3 sets
8 reps
p. 106

9
1–3 sets
8 reps
p. 95

10
1–3 sets
8 reps
p. 94

11
1–3 sets
8 reps
each arm
p. 94

12
1 set
10 reps
p. 104

Photocopy this page and take it with you when you work out.

FINE TUNING: BACK

This is a program of stretches and weight lifting exercises for overall body flexibility and strength, with special emphasis on the back.

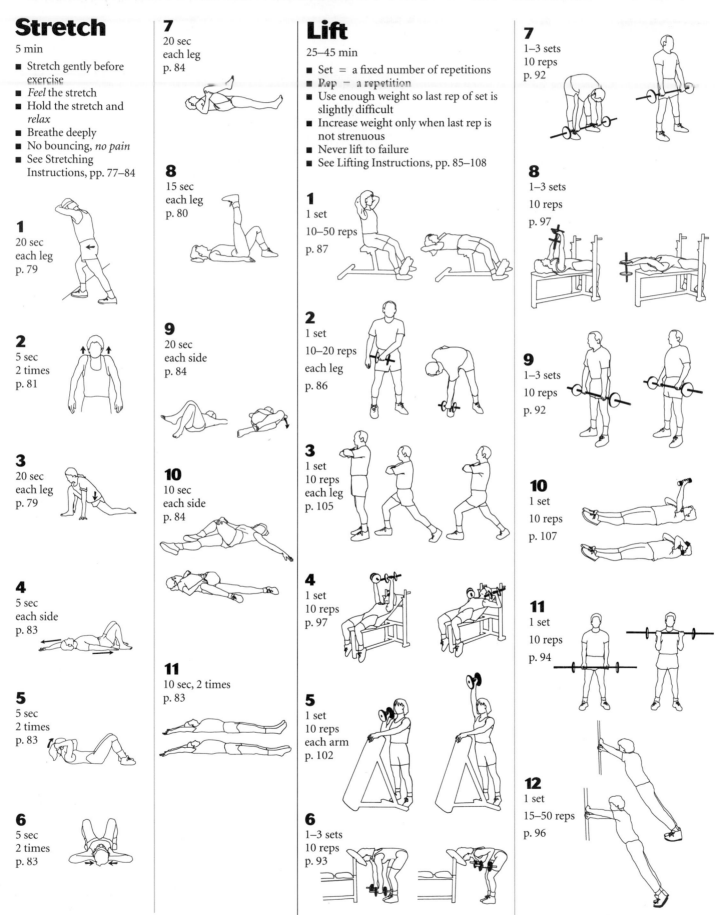

Stretch

5 min

- Stretch gently before exercise
- *Feel* the stretch
- Hold the stretch and *relax*
- Breathe deeply
- No bouncing, *no pain*
- See Stretching Instructions, pp. 77–84

1
20 sec
each leg
p. 79

2
5 sec
2 times
p. 81

3
20 sec
each leg
p. 79

4
5 sec
each side
p. 83

5
5 sec
2 times
p. 83

6
5 sec
2 times
p. 83

7
20 sec
each leg
p. 84

8
15 sec
each leg
p. 80

9
20 sec
each side
p. 84

10
10 sec
each side
p. 84

11
10 sec, 2 times
p. 83

Lift

25–45 min

- Set = a fixed number of repetitions
- Rep = a repetition
- Use enough weight so last rep of set is slightly difficult
- Increase weight only when last rep is not strenuous
- Never lift to failure
- See Lifting Instructions, pp. 85–108

1
1 set
10–50 reps
p. 87

2
1 set
10–20 reps
each leg
p. 86

3
1 set
10 reps
each leg
p. 105

4
1 set
10 reps
p. 97

5
1 set
10 reps
each arm
p. 102

6
1–3 sets
10 reps
p. 93

7
1–3 sets
10 reps
p. 92

8
1–3 sets
10 reps
p. 97

9
1–3 sets
10 reps
p. 92

10
1 set
10 reps
p. 107

11
1 set
10 reps
p. 94

12
1 set
15–50 reps
p. 96

Photocopy this page and take it with you when you work out.

FINE TUNING: BUTTOCKS

This is a program of stretches and weight lifting exercises for overall body flexibility and strength, with special emphasis on the buttocks.

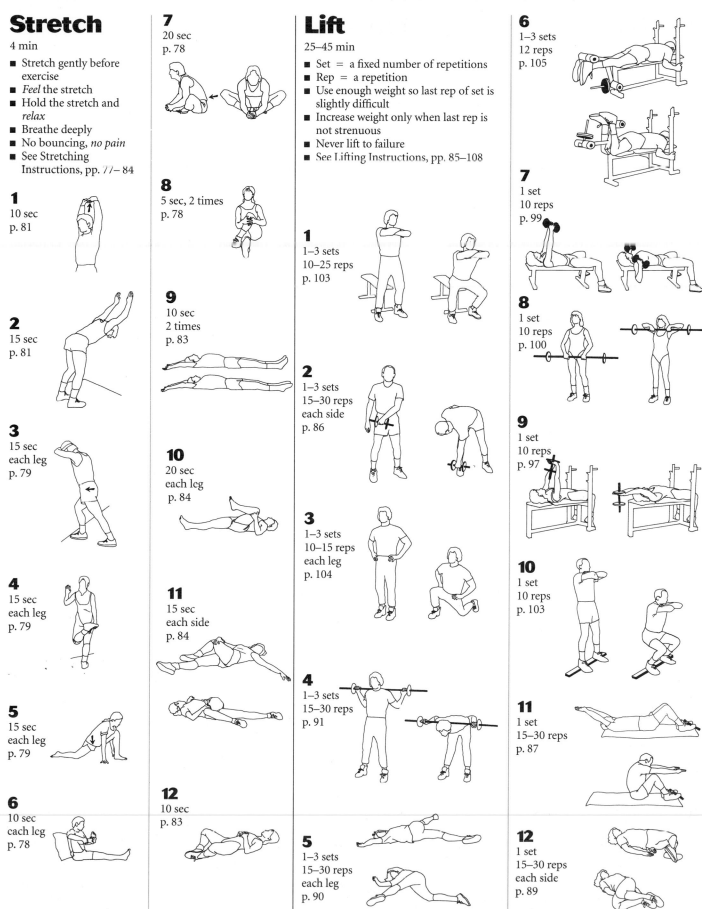

Stretch

4 min

- Stretch gently before exercise
- *Feel* the stretch
- Hold the stretch and *relax*
- Breathe deeply
- No bouncing, *no pain*
- See Stretching Instructions, pp. 77–84

1
10 sec
p. 81

2
15 sec
p. 81

3
15 sec
each leg
p. 79

4
15 sec
each leg
p. 79

5
15 sec
each leg
p. 79

6
10 sec
each leg
p. 78

7
20 sec
p. 78

8
5 sec, 2 times
p. 78

9
10 sec
2 times
p. 83

10
20 sec
each leg
p. 84

11
15 sec
each side
p. 84

12
10 sec
p. 83

Lift

25–45 min

- Set = a fixed number of repetitions
- Rep = a repetition
- Use enough weight so last rep of set is slightly difficult
- Increase weight only when last rep is not strenuous
- Never lift to failure
- See Lifting Instructions, pp. 85–108

1
1–3 sets
10–25 reps
p. 103

2
1–3 sets
15–30 reps
each side
p. 86

3
1–3 sets
10–15 reps
each leg
p. 104

4
1–3 sets
15–30 reps
p. 91

5
1–3 sets
15–30 reps
each leg
p. 90

6
1–3 sets
12 reps
p. 105

7
1 set
10 reps
p. 99

8
1 set
10 reps
p. 100

9
1 set
10 reps
p. 97

10
1 set
10 reps
p. 103

11
1 set
15–30 reps
p. 87

12
1 set
15–30 reps
each side
p. 89

Photocopy this page and take it with you when you work out.

FINE TUNING: CALVES

This is a program of stretches and weight lifting exercises for overall body flexibility and strength, with special emphasis on the calves.

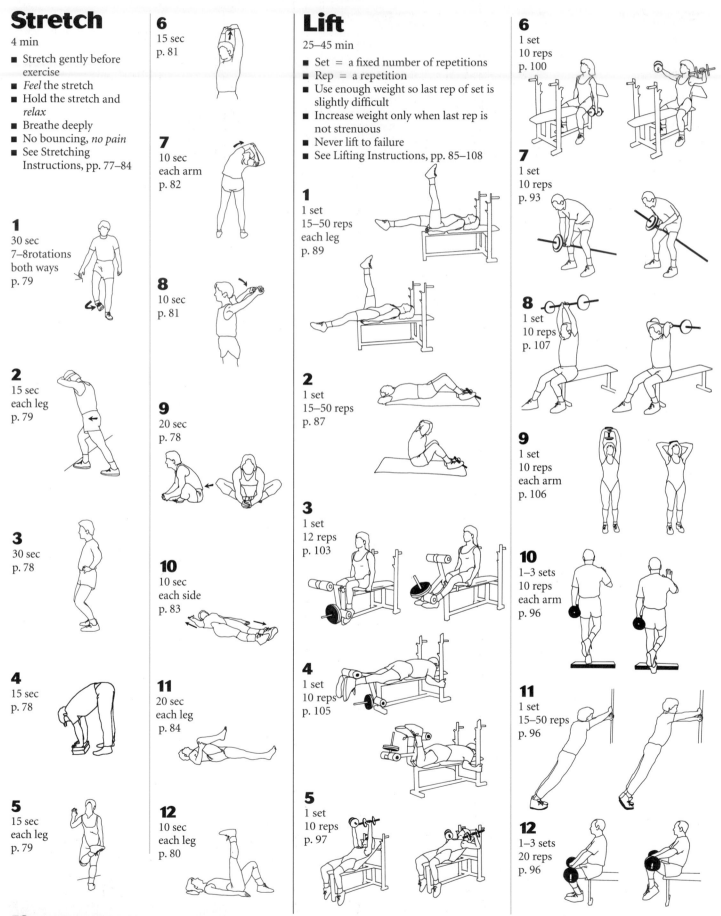

Stretch

4 min

- Stretch gently before exercise
- *Feel* the stretch
- Hold the stretch and *relax*
- Breathe deeply
- No bouncing, *no pain*
- See Stretching Instructions, pp. 77–84

1
30 sec
7–8 rotations
both ways
p. 79

2
15 sec
each leg
p. 79

3
30 sec
p. 78

4
15 sec
p. 78

5
15 sec
each leg
p. 79

6
15 sec
p. 81

7
10 sec
each arm
p. 82

8
10 sec
p. 81

9
20 sec
p. 78

10
10 sec
each side
p. 83

11
20 sec
each leg
p. 84

12
10 sec
each leg
p. 80

Lift

25–45 min

- Set = a fixed number of repetitions
- Rep = a repetition
- Use enough weight so last rep of set is slightly difficult
- Increase weight only when last rep is not strenuous
- Never lift to failure
- See Lifting Instructions, pp. 85–108

1
1 set
15–50 reps
each leg
p. 89

2
1 set
15–50 reps
p. 87

3
1 set
12 reps
p. 103

4
1 set
10 reps
p. 105

5
1 set
10 reps
p. 97

6
1 set
10 reps
p. 100

7
1 set
10 reps
p. 93

8
1 set
10 reps
p. 107

9
1 set
10 reps
each arm
p. 106

10
1–3 sets
10 reps
each arm
p. 96

11
1 set
15–50 reps
p. 96

12
1–3 sets
20 reps
p. 96

Photocopy this page and take it with you when you work out.

FINE TUNING: CHEST

This is a program of stretches and weight lifting exercises for overall body flexibility and strength, with special emphasis on the chest.

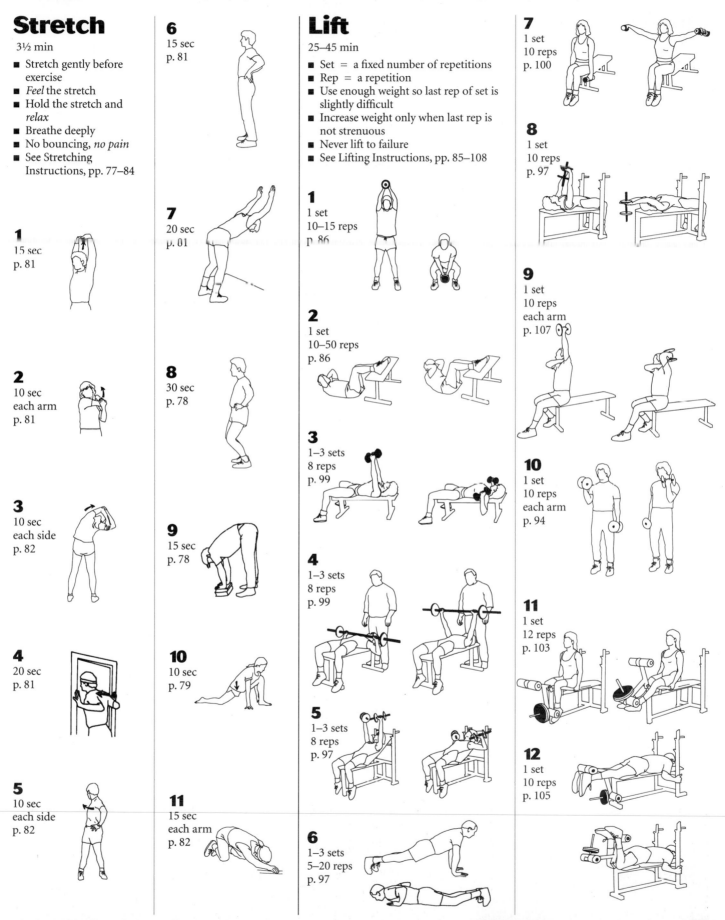

Stretch

3½ min

- Stretch gently before exercise
- *Feel* the stretch
- Hold the stretch and *relax*
- Breathe deeply
- No bouncing, *no pain*
- See Stretching Instructions, pp. 77–84

1
15 sec
p. 81

2
10 sec
each arm
p. 81

3
10 sec
each side
p. 82

4
20 sec
p. 81

5
10 sec
each side
p. 82

6
15 sec
p. 81

7
20 sec
p. 81

8
30 sec
p. 78

9
15 sec
p. 78

10
10 sec
p. 79

11
15 sec
each arm
p. 82

Lift

25–45 min

- Set = a fixed number of repetitions
- Rep = a repetition
- Use enough weight so last rep of set is slightly difficult
- Increase weight only when last rep is not strenuous
- Never lift to failure
- See Lifting Instructions, pp. 85–108

1
1 set
10–15 reps
p. 86

2
1 set
10–50 reps
p. 86

3
1–3 sets
8 reps
p. 99

4
1–3 sets
8 reps
p. 99

5
1–3 sets
8 reps
p. 97

6
1–3 sets
5–20 reps
p. 97

7
1 set
10 reps
p. 100

8
1 set
10 reps
p. 97

9
1 set
10 reps
each arm
p. 107

10
1 set
10 reps
each arm
p. 94

11
1 set
12 reps
p. 103

12
1 set
10 reps
p. 105

FINE TUNING: LEGS

This is a program of stretches and weight lifting exercises for overall body flexibility and strength, with special emphasis on the legs.

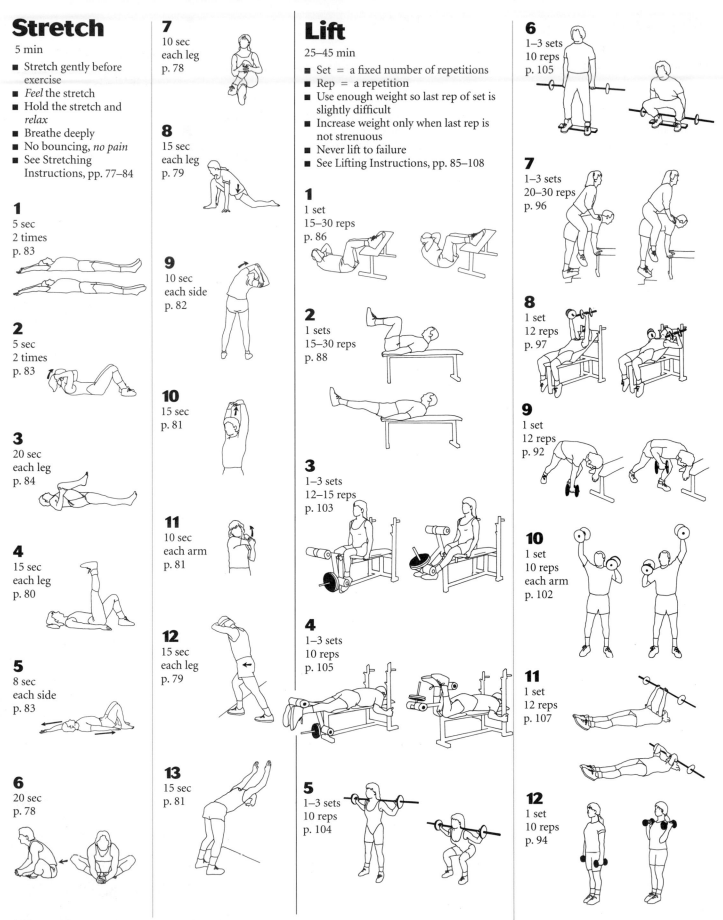

Stretch

5 min

- Stretch gently before exercise
- *Feel* the stretch
- Hold the stretch and *relax*
- Breathe deeply
- No bouncing, *no pain*
- See Stretching Instructions, pp. 77–84

1
5 sec
2 times
p. 83

2
5 sec
2 times
p. 83

3
20 sec
each leg
p. 84

4
15 sec
each leg
p. 80

5
8 sec
each side
p. 83

6
20 sec
p. 78

7
10 sec
each leg
p. 78

8
15 sec
each leg
p. 79

9
10 sec
each side
p. 82

10
15 sec
p. 81

11
10 sec
each arm
p. 81

12
15 sec
each leg
p. 79

13
15 sec
p. 81

Lift

25–45 min

- Set = a fixed number of repetitions
- Rep = a repetition
- Use enough weight so last rep of set is slightly difficult
- Increase weight only when last rep is not strenuous
- Never lift to failure
- See Lifting Instructions, pp. 85–108

1
1 set
15–30 reps
p. 86

2
1 sets
15–30 reps
p. 88

3
1–3 sets
12–15 reps
p. 103

4
1–3 sets
10 reps
p. 105

5
1–3 sets
10 reps
p. 104

6
1–3 sets
10 reps
p. 105

7
1–3 sets
20–30 reps
p. 96

8
1 set
12 reps
p. 97

9
1 set
12 reps
p. 92

10
1 set
10 reps
each arm
p. 102

11
1 set
12 reps
p. 107

12
1 set
10 reps
p. 94

Photocopy this page and take it with you when you work out.

FINE TUNING: SHOULDERS

This is a program of stretches and weight lifting exercises for overall body flexibility and strength, with special emphasis on the shoulders.

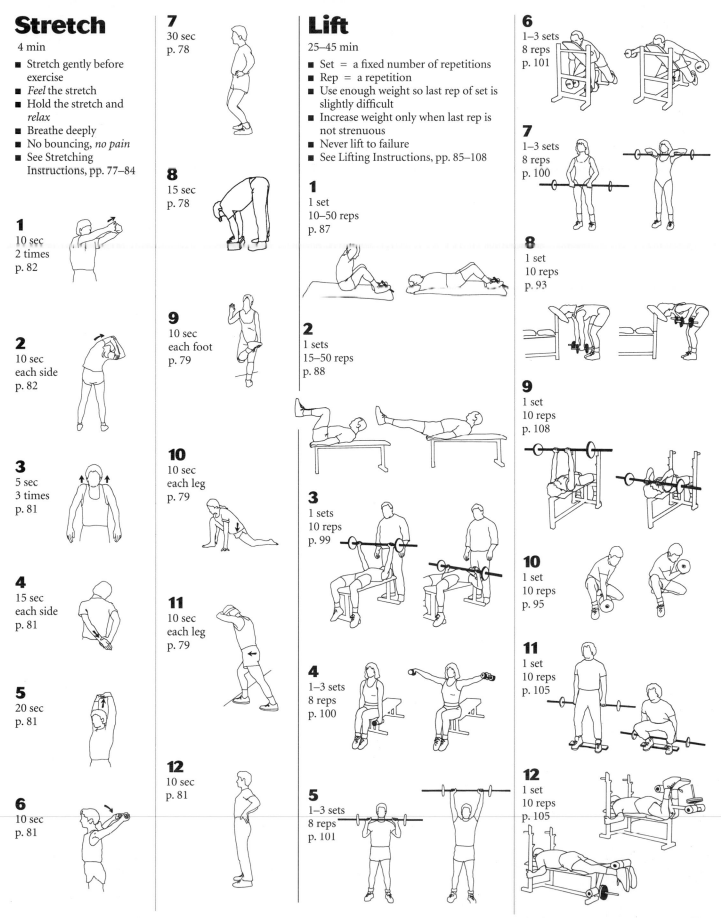

Stretch

4 min

- Stretch gently before exercise
- *Feel* the stretch
- Hold the stretch and *relax*
- Breathe deeply
- No bouncing, *no pain*
- See Stretching Instructions, pp. 77–84

1
10 sec
2 times
p. 82

2
10 sec
each side
p. 82

3
5 sec
3 times
p. 81

4
15 sec
each side
p. 81

5
20 sec
p. 81

6
10 sec
p. 81

7
30 sec
p. 78

8
15 sec
p. 78

9
10 sec
each foot
p. 79

10
10 sec
each leg
p. 79

11
10 sec
each leg
p. 79

12
10 sec
p. 81

Lift

25–45 min

- Set = a fixed number of repetitions
- Rep = a repetition
- Use enough weight so last rep of set is slightly difficult
- Increase weight only when last rep is not strenuous
- Never lift to failure
- See Lifting Instructions, pp. 85–108

1
1 set
10–50 reps
p. 87

2
1 sets
15–50 reps
p. 88

3
1 sets
10 reps
p. 99

4
1–3 sets
8 reps
p. 100

5
1–3 sets
8 reps
p. 101

6
1–3 sets
8 reps
p. 101

7
1–3 sets
8 reps
p. 100

8
1 set
10 reps
p. 93

9
1 set
10 reps
p. 108

10
1 set
10 reps
p. 95

11
1 set
10 reps
p. 105

12
1 set
10 reps
p. 105

Photocopy this page and take it with you when you work out.

3 THE INSTRUCTIONS

There are three basic components to getting in shape:

- **Moving**
- **Stretching**
- **Lifting**

For all three activities there are *general* instructions.

For each stretch and weight training exercise, there are *specific* instructions.

CROSS REFERENCE

Under each stretch and exercise in every program is a page number from this section of instructions. When doing any stretch or exercise for the first time, turn to the page number listed. After a while, you'll know what to do and will only need to use this section when performing a new stretch or exercise.

For any moving exercise you are not familiar with, read the general instructions here before starting. Even if you've done the activity before (you've certainly walked, for example), you may still find some interesting tips that will help you along the way.

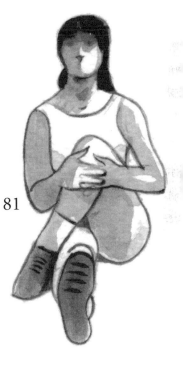

MOVING

STRETCHING

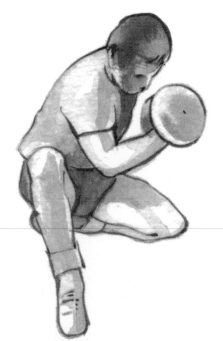

LIFTING

HOW TO MOVE

Here are some ideas for improving the effectiveness of your walking, cycling, swimming, or running. Remember, you are not limited to these activities — you needn't always put on a sweatsuit and pound down the pavement to improve your cardiovascular fitness. There's tennis and golf, ping pong, basketball, and jumping rope. What's important is that you *move.* Do something, whenever you can, to get your heart pumping harder.

Measuring your heart rate is a good way to tell how hard you're working your heart. It's especially important if you haven't exercised for a while. Measure your heart rate when you start exercising, whether you're doing typical athletic activities, such as walking, running, cycling, or swimming, or working in the garden, cutting wood, shoveling snow, or dancing.

HEART RATE

See p. 117 for specific directions on how to check your heart rate.

- *Program Before the Program.* Don't worry about heart rate if you are following these programs, since you will be exercising at such a moderate level. Just don't get uncomfortably out of breath.

- *Basic Programs 1–5.* Here, you'll want to start checking your heart rate so you understand how your heart responds to exercise. Exercise at a comfortable rate, checking your pulse and comparing it to your maximum heart rate. Don't worry about percentages at first.

- *After you get in better shape,* a reasonable zone would be 50% of maximum or higher.

PERCEIVED EXERTION METHOD

RULE OF THUMB

You should be able to carry on a conversation while exercising.

This is an intuitive, rather than a scientific method. After you check your pulse for a while, you'll be able to tell from your own breathing how hard you're working. You'll be able to sense when you're exercising hard enough to get a training effect. For example, if you decide to exercise at 50% of your maximum heart rate, take your pulse and concentrate on how this level *feels.* Many factors will go into this, such as how you feel that day, the condition you're in, the heat, headwinds, etc., all of which can be measured by how out-of-breath you are. After you practice this sensitivity for a while, you'll be able to make a close-enough guess of a 50% rate without taking your pulse or counting.

LONGER WORKOUT/LOWER INTENSITY

Many people prefer longer, slower workouts. (By "longer" we're referring to the times indicated in the Programs.) You might enjoy longer, more relaxed workouts, at a lower pulse rate. The benefits can be the same. Feel free to experiment.

EFFECT OF MEDICATIONS ON HEART RATE

See pp. 165–167 on high blood pressure.

Certain types of medication do affect your heart rate; for example, the class of drugs known as beta blockers (often prescribed for high blood pressure or chest pains) lower your heart rate. Many other medications affect heart rate (tranquilizers, diet and thyroid medications, bronchodilators, etc.), so if you are taking anything, check with your doctor.

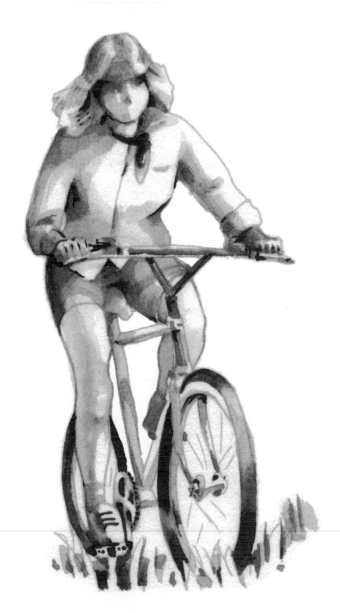

In the last few years, walking has become the most popular form of exercise in America. Over 55 million Americans list walking as their major fitness activity. Why such popularity? For one thing, it's the simplest form of aerobic exercise. Everyone knows how to do it, it can be done any time of day, you don't need specialized equipment (other than a good pair of shoes), it's inexpensive and suitable for any age group. Also, literally millions of people have found — from trial and error — that it doesn't entail the overexertion or injuries common in many other activities, such as running.

QUICK WALKS

When you're busy:

- Walk during your lunch hour. Or walk *to* lunch. Or do some errands at lunch time.

- Take a walk break instead of a coffee break.

- Park the car in the farthest corner of the parking lot and walk to your destination.

- Set up a walk-and-talk instead of a sit-and-talk appointment or date.

- Walk to see a friend or coworker in the office instead of phoning.

- Walk with the kids when babysitting.

- Take a five-minute walk whenever you can.

THE ELEMENTS OF STYLE

No two people walk quite the same way. Your style of walking is as individual as your fingerprints.

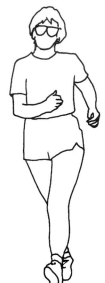

- Stretch before and after walking. The heel-to-toe action of walking tends to tighten your calf muscles, so stretching the lower legs is important.

- Start *slowly* at a comfortable pace.

- Maintain *good posture*. Keep ears centered over shoulders, which should be centered over hips. Don't slump. Keep your chest up and out and shoulders relaxed. With this posture there will be less chance of foot, leg, or back pain.

- *Heel first, rock,* then swing the foot forward. Sounds simple, but as you walk faster it's harder to maintain the rocking motion. Keep your foot swing natural.

- *Pace yourself.* Use the target heart rate *(see pp. 117–118)* to set your pace. Walking at a moderate rate will increase your stamina.

- Don't forget to *swing your arms.*

WALKING PROGRAM A TEN WEEK PROGRAM FOR BEGINNERS

1st week	stretch 5 min	walk ¼ mile a day	stretch 5 min
2nd week	stretch 5 min	walk ½ mile a day	stretch 5 min
3rd week	stretch 5 min	walk ¾ mile a day	stretch 5 min
4th week	stretch 5 min	walk 1 mile a day	stretch 5 min
5th week	stretch 5 min	walk 1 mile a day	stretch 5 min
6th week	stretch 5 min	walk 1 mile a day	stretch 5 min
7th week	stretch 5 min	walk 1¼ miles a day	stretch 5 min
8th week	stretch 5 min	walk 1½ miles a day	stretch 5 min
9th week	stretch 5 min	walk 1¾ miles a day	stretch 5 min
10th week	stretch 5 min	walk 2 miles a day	stretch 5 min

WALKING

MALL WALKING

Believe it or not, there are some three million mall walkers in the United States. It's an especially popular activity with older people. Malls are relatively safe and almost always weatherproof. And there are no curbs, hills, or gutters. Many people go mall walking in small groups — it's a means of socializing while exercising.

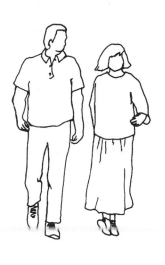

FITNESS FROM WALKING

The Institute for Aerobics Research (*see Further Reading, below*) recommends the following:

MINIMUM DOSE FOR MODERATE FITNESS

Women: Walk 2 miles in 30 min or less 3 days a week *or* walk 2 miles in 30–40 min 5–6 days a week.
Men: Walk 2 miles in 27 min or less at least 3 days a week *or* walk 2 miles in 30–40 min 6–7 days a week.

MIMIMUM DOSE FOR HIGH FITNESS

Women: Walk 2 miles in 30 min 5–6 days a week *or* run 2 miles in 20–24 min 4 days a week.
Men: Walk 2.5 miles in 38 min 6–7 days a week *or* run 2 miles in 20 min or less 4–5 days a week.

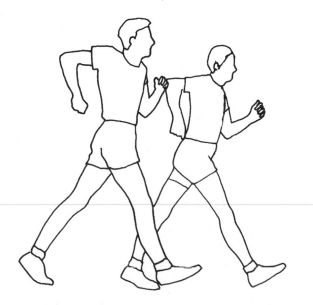

THESE SHOES ARE MADE FOR WALKIN'

Great strides (sic) have been made in walking shoes in the last decade. *Walking Medicine (see reference below)* has an excellent section, "The Walking Shoe and Foot Book." A good running shoe store with a knowledgeable staff can give you advice. Or look at a current issue of *Walking* magazine.

What to look for in a walking shoe:

- An extra-flexible sole to accommodate the greater bending of serious walking.
- Good shock absorption, especially at the heel, yet firm enough for stability.
- Adequate arch support.
- A permeable top that lets air circulate and moisture escape.

CALORIES BURNED BY WALKING ONE HOUR

SPEED (MPH)	WEIGHT 120 lb	160 lb	200 lb
2	160	210	265
3	215	285	360
4	280	375	470

FURTHER READING

Walking Handbook © 1989. Institute for Aerobics Research, 12330 Preston Road, Dallas, TX 75230.

Walking Medicine: The Lifetime Guide to Preventive and Therapeutic Exercisewalking Programs © 1990 by Gary Yanker and Kathy Burton. McGraw-Hill, NY.

Dr. James M. Rippe's Complete Book of Fitness Walking © 1990 by James M. Rippe, M.D., and Ann Ward, Ph.D. Prentice Hall, NY.

Walking magazine, monthly. 9-11 Harcourt St., Boston, MA 02116.

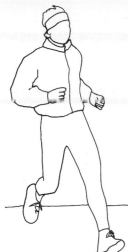

If walking is such an excellent fitness activity, why go faster? Because jogging and running are just extensions of walking, and will add intensity to your program. Running also takes less time for the same aerobic and calorie-burning benefits. One major benefit of jogging and running is often overlooked: because your bones and joints get more pressure exerted on them, they grow stronger and this affords better protection against osteoporosis (the deterioration of bones that occurs with aging).

Jogging, like walking, is one of the best aerobic activities. You don't need special equipment (like a bike), or facilities (like a pool). And jogging is easier to master than cycling, swimming, cross-country skiing, tennis, or other ball sports.

JOGGING VS. RUNNING

Just what is the difference between jogging and running? Joggers move at a slower speed and rarely enter races; most people moving at a pace of 9 or 10 minutes per mile or faster call themselves runners. Whether you call yourself a jogger or a runner, the key is to exercise at a pace that feels comfortable for you and at the same time provides you with aerobic benefits.

With increased intensity comes increased risk of injury. Jogging and running can place added stress on your hips, legs, and feet. But if you warm up and stretch, use good shoes, and avoid overtraining, you will be able to avoid injuries. As with weight training, a day of rest is useful. If you are at all concerned with injuries, only run every other day. Listen to your body. If it rebels, respond accordingly.

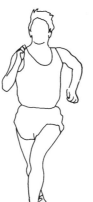

GET OFF ON THE RIGHT FOOT

The only equipment you'll need are good shoes. Find a running shoe store where the sales people are runners. Go in late afternoon when your feet tend to be slightly swollen. Take a pair of athletic socks.

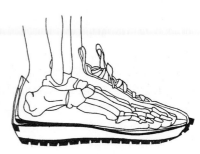

Look for good cushioning, ample toe room, and snug heel fit. The shoe should feel like an extension of your foot. Take a spin down the pavement outside the store. Any serious running shoe store will allow you to do this.

STARTING TO RUN

- Walk before you run. Keep at it until you can walk easily for 20 to 30 min.

- Next, walk briskly until you can do so for 20 to 30 min.

- Now do some jogging — not for the whole distance, but jog for 100 yards or so 3 to 4 times during your brisk walk.

- Increase the jogging, and eventually begin to run. Keep things comfortable. Take it slow.

- Maybe you'll feel more comfortable jogging than running. Or maybe you'll run, with periods of jogging — go by your heart rate and how you feel.

WATER RUNNING

Some years ago, injured runners discovered that running in water enabled them to continue training while injuries healed. You might want to use a flotation device made especially for this purpose. Or a life jacket from an Army-Navy store. The idea is to get in deep water and exercise your legs in a running motion as you would on land. The water provides resistance, but without the impact of land running that aggravates injuries. Stay upright, and don't lean too far forward. Keep your elbows close to your body. It may help to keep palms open as you move your arms, for balance.

RUNNING WITH HAND WEIGHTS

We do not recommend carrying weights in your hands or on your ankles while running, although the practice is okay when walking. Hand weights *can* strengthen the upper body, but they'll also slow you down and reduce aerobic gains overall.

But the main reason we discourage this practice is the increased risk of injury: the more weight, the greater impact for each footstrike. Hand weights are notorious for injuring knees. You can get just as good an upper body workout with less risk using a pair of dumbbells in the gym in a very short time.

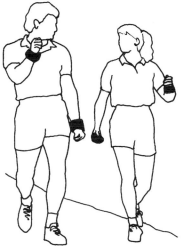

RUNNING DOESN'T ACCELERATE ARTHRITIS

Several studies on active people, including runners, show their chance of developing arthritis is the same as in sedentary people. Exercise is good for joints, and even the pounding from years of running doesn't increase arthritis risk. A recent study at the University of California in San Francisco and Stanford University goes even further. Running doesn't even increase the rate of knee deterioration in runners who have arthritis.

FURTHER READING

Galloway's Book on Running by Jeff Galloway © 1984. Shelter Publications, Bolinas, CA.

Runner's World Magazine. Monthly. Rodale Press, 33 E. Minor St., Emmaus, PA 18098.

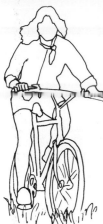

Cycling is another activity that's greatly increased in popularity recently. People of all ages enjoy it. It's one of the greatest cardiovascular activities and it places very little stress on the joints. Plus, there are aesthetic fringe benefits: picture yourself cycling down the road, feeling the wind, taking in beautiful scenery.

THE RIGHT BIKE

Shop wisely for a bicycle. It's important to find the bike that's right for *you.* The basic recreational bike has 10 to 24 speeds, dropped handlebars (which can be replaced by upright ones), a light alloy frame, and alloy wheels.

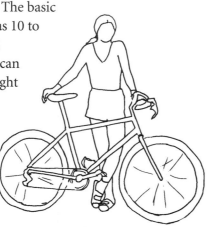

Mountain bikes have wider tires and upright handlebars; most have 18 to 24 speeds. These bikes were originally designed for off-road riding, but cyclists have learned that they work equally well on the roads and especially in cities, where there may be holes in the pavement or curbs to contend with. If you especially want to ride some off-road trails, a mountain bike may be your best bet.

BIKE FIT

Nothing is better than an experienced, honest bike salesperson, but here are a few rules of thumb:

- *Frame size:* When you stand directly over the bike, the top tube should be about 2 to 3 inches lower than your crotch.

- *Seat height:* With your shoes on, your knee should be slightly bent when that leg is at the bottom of the pedaling stroke.

- *Handlebars:* Width should be equal to your shoulder width. Height of handlebar stems (the piece that attaches the handlebars to the frame) should be 1 to 1¼ inches below the top of the seat.

STREET RIDING

Newcomers to cycling often ask, "How do you find a good, relatively safe cycling route?"
Riding on most town and city streets is enjoyable and safe if a few simple rules are followed. You won't be intimidated by cars if you know that the secret to safe, confident riding is to become a natural part of the traffic flow.

First, gain confidence in basic bike handling skills, so you can shift gears, stop smoothly, turn rapidly, and scan quickly for traffic. Learn to do all these things without swerving. Practice makes perfect, and empty parking lots or quiet residential streets are good places to improve these skills.

PEDAL REVOLUTIONS PER MINUTE

Work on developing proper pedal technique. Learn how to increase cadence (pedal revolutions per minute) into the 70 to 90 range: 70 means 70 downstrokes of your right foot (full revolutions of the pedal) in one minute. Being in the right gear will vary according to terrain. Practice changing gears, learning which ones are right for your cadence. Don't use too high a gear, which strains your knees.

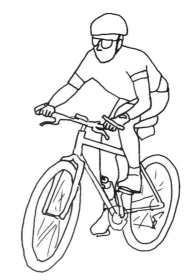

CYCLING

HEAD FIRST

Always wear a helmet.

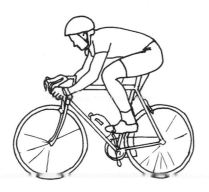

Never wear a Walkman. (You can't hear warning sounds, such as a car approaching too close.)

CROSS TRAINING

Cycling can be a great activity for improving your performance in other sports. Runners use cycling because it develops different leg muscles (especially quadriceps) than does running. Cycling is excellent for swimmers, who mostly use their arms. In improving the strength of your legs, cycling allows you to increase your cardiovascular fitness, and can work to balance other aerobic activities.

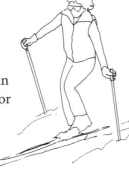

STATIONARY CYCLING

Exercycles have the same aerobic benefits as outdoor cycling, but can be used indoors at any time of day or night, when the weather's too cold outside. Using these machines provides a quick and practical way to get a good aerobic workout in a very short time. Some people watch the evening news while doing a 30-minute exercycle workout. In some health clubs you can see a bank of people on exercycles (often the computerized

Lifecycles), reading the morning paper — getting their day's aerobic workout and catching up on the news before going to work.

Another device that has become popular in recent years is the "wind load" simulator. Here you remove the front wheel from your bike and place your bike on to the simulator. There is usually a small roller that the rear wheel turns on and two squirrel-cage attachments that provide tension as you pedal.

CALORIES BURNED CYCLING

MPH	CALORIES BURNED PER MINUTE
5.5	4.5
9.4	7.0
13.1	11.1

FURTHER READING

Fitness Cycling by Chris Carmichael and Edmund R. Burke © 1994. Human Kinetics Publishers, Champaign, IL.

The All-New Complete Book of Cycling by Eugene A. Sloane © 1988. Simon & Schuster, New York.

Bicycling Magazine's New Bike Owner's Guide by Bicycling Magazine Editors © 1990. Rodale Press, Emmaus, PA.

Cycling, Health and Physiology by Edmund R. Burke © 1992. Vitresse Press, Brattleboro, VT.

Bicycling magazine. Monthly. 33 E. Minor St., Emmaus, PA 18098.

Bicycle Guide. Monthly. 1415 Third St., Suite 303, Santa Monica, CA, 90401.

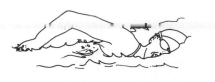

If you ask anyone which sport provides the best overall body workout, the answer will most likely be swimming. Is this right and if so, just how does swimming go about building a strong, fit body?

THE ADVANTAGES OF SWIMMING

- Swimming uses most of the body's major muscle groups, especially if you do various strokes. The motion of your arms and legs against the resistance of the water works the muscles of the arms, shoulders, hips, abdominals, and legs. Moving all your major joints through a wide range of motion improves flexibility, as well as range of motion.

- Swimming is beneficial if you are overweight or have joint problems that keep you from other aerobic activities, or are pregnant or getting back in shape after childbirth.

- Your body weighs less in the water than it does on land and this cushioning effect means you can get a very good workout without pounding your lower limbs, decreasing risk of injuries.

- Swimming is an excellent activity for burning calories. As you get in shape and improve your stroke mechanics, your speed and endurance will increase. You can expect to burn in the range of 600 to 800 calories per hour swimming, depending on which stroke you use.

- Swimming is a great summertime activity if you live in a hot or humid environment. Cool water is refreshing on a hot summer's day.

ANY DRAWBACKS?

Swimming is an ideal form of exercise, but it's not perfect.

- First, you need a place to swim. Unless you live in southern states, you'll have to rely on an indoor pool most of the year.

- Second, if you are a nonswimmer or need work on your technique, you'll want to take lessons before you consider using swimming to improve your fitness and health.

But these obstacles are not insurmountable.

If you have (or want to prevent) osteoporosis, weight bearing activities will be a better choice than swimming. Walking or jogging stimulates bone strength through impact, which is absent in swimming.

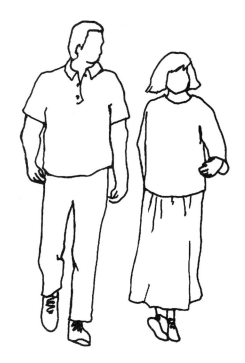

SWIMMING

DIFFERENT STROKES

The freestyle, or crawl, is the best stroke for cardio-vascular benefit. Little energy is wasted here, and the freestyle's steady, rhythmic movements maximize heart and lung benefits and burn calories. The other strokes, in order of aerobic benefits are backstroke, breaststroke, and sidestroke. Use various strokes for variety and pleasure.

SWIMNASTICS

Swimnastics are exercises done in the water. Many common calisthenic and flexibility exercises can be modified for the water. Swimnastics has become increasingly popular, especially for older people, or those with weak muscles or joint problems, because it is less stressful for the joints and muscles than many other activities. Its cardiovascular benefits may not be as great as other aerobic activities, but it makes a good starting point, and is an excellent warmup before swimming laps. Check with your local health club, YMCA, or neighborhood pool for classes. It's sociable and stimulating.

WATER WALKING

Walking in water is an excellent way to burn calories and lose weight. You stride through the water, usually thigh-deep or deeper. The deeper the water, the more calories burned. In deep water you can get an upper body workout by swinging your arms against the water's resistance. This can be done at the beach or in a pool. For variety, walk sideways, backwards, and forward. Try some aerobic dance steps. Keep moving. *(See Water Running, p. 69.)*

FURTHER READING

Total Swimming by Harvey S. Wiener © 1980. Fireside/Simon & Schuster, New York, NY.

Swim for Fitness by Marianne Brems © 1985. Chronicle Books, San Francisco, CA.

Water Workout: 120 Water Exercises For Swimmers and Nonswimmers by Bill Reed and Murray Rose © 1986. Crown Books/Random House, New York, NY.

The Water Workout Recovery Program by Robert G. Watkins © 1988. Contemporary Books, Chicago, IL.

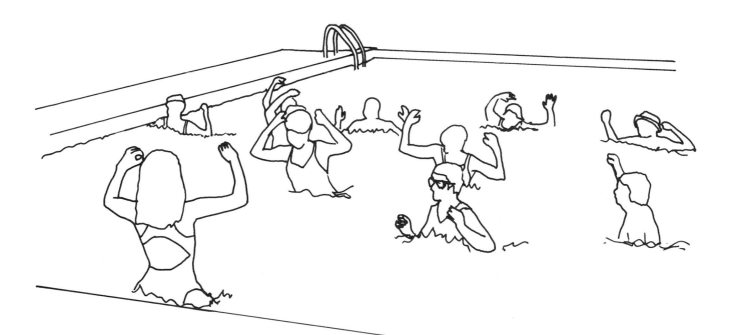

HOW TO MOVE

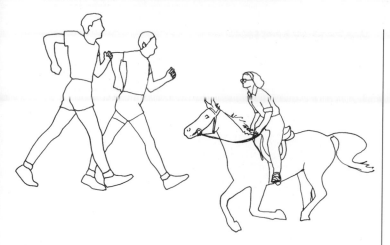

Aerobic means "with oxygen." Any activity that increases your heart rate and circulation can be termed *aerobic exercise.* Typical aerobic exercises are distance running, cycling, swimming, cross-country skiing — those that use large muscle groups. Walking can also provide aerobic exercise.

AEROBIC VARIETY

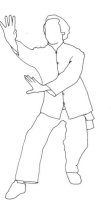

You don't *have* to run, cycle, or swim to get aerobic exercise. Anything that gets your heart rate up qualifies. There are many activities not normally thought of as "aerobic" that can increase heart rate. Think of putting a little extra effort into say, cutting the lawn, or vacuuming the house, or washing the car. Any physical activity can be made (more) aerobic.

CLASSES

Classes provide great motivation. All you have to do is show up and you know you'll get a workout. And exercising in a roomful of other people can be inspiring — all that energy rubs off!

Aerobic dance classes are available in a "low-impact" format, with music providing the backbeat. Other "ancient" forms of exercise, such as yoga, tai chi, and chi gung, will teach you how to stretch, direct your breath and/or increase your "chi," or life force.

EXERCISE MACHINES

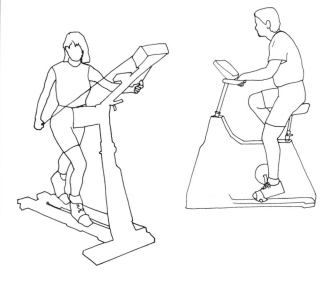

There is a great variety of exercise machines designed to get your heart rate up. Most health clubs stock a wall of them, and many are available for home use. These include treadmills, stair-steppers, stationary bikes, cross-country skiing and rowing machines. As opposed to the Universal, Nautilus or Soloflex systems, which use weight resistance, these machines, while exercising and strengthening the muscles, also provide aerobic benefits.

FURTHER READING

Aerobics by Kenneth H. Cooper© 1992. Bantam, New York, NY.

Living with Exercise © 1991 by Steven Blair. American Health Publishing Co., Dallas, TX.

Fitness Without Exercise by Bryant A. Stamford, Ph.D. and Porter Shimer © 1990. Warner Books, New York, NY.

ACSM Fitness Book, American College of Sports Medicine © 1992. Human Kinetics Publishers, Champaign, IL.

SPORTS

Sports are fun, social, good discipline, and provide excellent health benefits. Team sports teach children and adults how to get along and work together, and how to win (or lose) gracefully. Your competitive nature may help you improve your athletic performance and skills, with the added side benefits of improved health. Solitary sports allow you to compete against your own "personal best." Goals are achievable, because you set them, and you improve at your own pace.

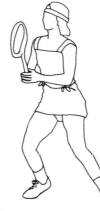

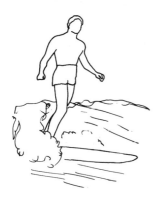

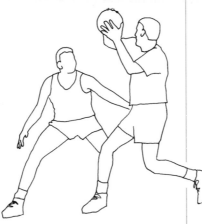

CROSS-COUNTRY SKIING

More and more people are discovering that cross-country skiing provides a way to combine physical activity and enjoyment of the wintery outdoors. Cross-country skiing provides you with an excellent complement to other programs of walking, running, or cycling. Not only does it give one of the better cardiovascular workouts of any exercise, skiing relieves the jarring of running and helps build upper body strength. This activity can be practiced both outdoors on groomed trails or indoors on a cross-country ski machine.

HOW TO MOVE

TENNIS

Bill Wright, Tennis Coach at the University of Arizona, invented a concept called *Aerobic Tennis*, where you maximize effort by:

- running as fast, as far, and as hard as you can
- moving away from the ball so you can step into it
- getting your heart pumping strongly to improve your cardiovascular fitness
- involving your *whole body* in every move
- working up a sweat to get the workout you've been looking for

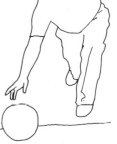

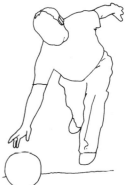

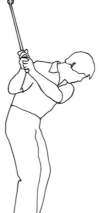

HOW TO MOVE

WHITE COLLAR EXERCISE

Even if you have a "sedentary" job, you can build exercise into the workday. See the *On the Job* and *Busy Day* sections (pp. 33–35 and 36–37) for recommended stretches and exercises.

YARDWORK

When you schedule the aerobic part of your Program, don't forget that work is a workout!

- Pushing a lawn mower uses as many calories as cycling. Some people are trading in their power mowers for old-fashioned human-powered ones. Burn calories instead of gasoline!

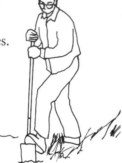

- Gardening can use almost as many calories as moderate swimming.

Your sense of accomplishment will be twofold: you get your exercise and the job done at the same time. Chop and stack the wood and then stand back and feel your biceps while you admire the symmetry of the woodpile. When you shovel snow, get your heart rate up. Make your work *more* of a workout.

BLUE COLLAR WORK

Any work that involves using your body will already be burning calories. Increased awareness of the way you lift and carry can help prevent injuries on the job, and keep you in good shape while you do good work.

- Always bend your knees when picking up heavy objects. Keep the weight on the hamstrings, which are large, strong muscles, instead of on your back.
- Stretch before and after your workday to keep muscles flexible and limber. Take mini stretching breaks in between tasks.
- Again, as with yardwork or housework, think of ways to strengthen your muscles from your work and even possibly get some cardiovascular benefits.

WORK AND PLAY

HOUSEWORK

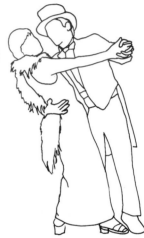

- Stretch a little farther as you lean across the mattress to make the bed.
- Push a broom instead of a vacuum cleaner.
- Pick up the pace; try getting your heart rate up as you move from chore to chore.
- Hang clothes outside and inhale deeply; be conscious of your breathing throughout the day.

PLAY

Walking your dog, taking a stroll with the baby in a backpack, playing Frisbee, and dancing are all forms of exercise that are enjoyable as well as aerobic. You might as well have a good time while you're at it; that alone makes your heart feel better. Yoga can be aerobic. Chi gung (the "internal energy development") is an ancient Chinese practice that uses meditation and body awareness to strengthen internal organs and improve overall health. Classes in chi gung are now becoming more widely available in America.

FURTHER READING

Living with Exercise by Steven N. Blair © 1991. American Health Publishers, Dallas, TX.

Biomarkers: The 10 Determinants of Aging You Can Control by William Evans and Irwin Rosenberg, © 1991. Simon & Schuster, New York, NY.

We Live Too Short and Die Too Young by Walter Bortz, © 1991. Bantam Books, New York, NY.

HOW TO STRETCH

Stretching is simple. But there is a right way and a wrong way to stretch. The right way is a slow, relaxed stretch while you focus on the muscles being stretched. The wrong way (practiced by many) is to bounce, or to push the stretch to the point of pain or beyond — these methods can do more harm than good.

THE EASY STRETCH   Stretch to the point where you feel a *mild tension*, then relax as you hold the stretch for 5 to 15 seconds. DO NOT BOUNCE! The feeling of tension should ease as you hold the stretch. If it doesn't, ease off slightly until things feel comfortable. The easy stretch reduces the muscular tightness and readies the muscles for the developmental stretch.

THE DEVELOPMENTAL STRETCH   Move slowly into the developmental stretch, a fraction of an inch farther until you feel mild tension and hold it for 5 to 15 seconds. No bouncing. Again, the tension should diminish. If it does not, ease off.

THE ONE-PHASE STRETCH   Doing just the easy stretch will release tension and make you feel better. It's valuable even without the developmental stretch. It helps you maintain your current flexibility.

BREATHING   Breathe slowly and naturally. Do not hold your breath while stretching.

RELAXATION   Keep the hands, feet, shoulders, and jaw relaxed as you stretch. Tension in these places will hinder your stretching.

THE STRETCH REFLEX   Whenever you stretch muscle fibers too far (either by bouncing or pushing too far), a nerve reflex signals the muscles to contract. This *stretch reflex* is one of the body's automatic defense mechanisms and keeps the muscles from being injured. When you overdo it, you tighten the very muscles you're trying to stretch.

A word of caution: pushing a stretch too far or bouncing can strain the muscles and activate the stretch reflex. If you stretch too far, you may cause microscopic damage to the muscle fibers. These small muscle tears lead to formation of scar tissue, with a gradual loss of elasticity.

NO PAIN, NO GAIN?   Pain is a sign something is *wrong*. Pay attention to it and back off! Most stretching injuries have come from people pushing too far or too fast.

WHAT'S THE RIGHT FEELING?   It should feel mild, not intense. It should feel like you can hold it indefinitely. We all have different levels of flexibility; don't compare yourself with others. Stretching isn't a contest. Everyone is different.

HOW TO STRETCH

LOWER BACK, HIPS, GROIN, AND HAMSTRINGS

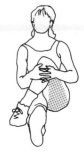

1

- Stand with feet shoulder-width apart
- Keep heels flat, toes pointed straight ahead
- Assume bent knee position (quarter squat)
- Hold 30 sec

Relaxes hamstrings, stretches calves, achilles, and ankles

2
- Stand with feet shoulder-width apart
- Keep heels flat, toes pointed straight ahead
- With knees slightly bent, bend forward at hips
- Keep arms and neck relaxed
- Hold 10 to 20 sec
- Do not lock knees or bounce
- Keep knees slightly bent as you return to upright position

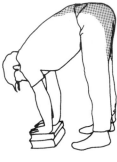

Stretches lower back and hamstrings

3
- Sit on floor, soles of feet together; hold onto toes and feet
- Gently pull forward bending from the hips
- Hold 10 to 30 sec
- Do not bounce
- Breathe slowly and deeply

Stretches lower back and groin

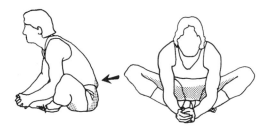

4
- Sit on floor with right leg straight out in front
- Bend left leg, cross left foot over, place outside right knee
- Pull left knee across body toward opposite shoulder
- Hold 10 to 20 sec
- Repeat on other side
- Breathe easily

Stretches side of hip, hamstrings

5
- Sit on floor with left leg straight out in front
- Bend right leg, cross right foot over, place outside left knee
- Bend left elbow and rest it outside right knee
- Place right hand behind hips on floor
- Turn head over right shoulder, rotate upper body right
- Hold 10 to 15 sec
- Repeat on other side
- Breathe slowly

Stretches lower back, side of hip, and neck

6
- Sit on floor with left leg straight out in front
- Hold onto outside of right ankle with left hand, with right hand and forearm around bent knee
- Gently pull leg as one unit toward chest until you feel easy stretch in back of upper leg; no stress at knee
- You may rest your back against something for support
- Hold 10 to 20 sec
- Repeat on other side

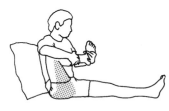

Stretches hamstrings and side of hip

LEGS

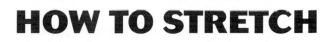

1

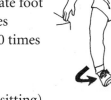

- Stand and hold onto something for balance
- Lift right foot and rotate foot and ankle 8 to 10 times clockwise, then 8 to 10 times counterclockwise
- Repeat on other side

(Note: can also be done sitting)

Stretches ankles

2

- Stand a little way from wall and lean on it with forearms, head resting on hands
- Place right foot in front of you, leg bent, left leg straight behind you
- Slowly move hips forward until you feel stretch in calf of left leg
- Keep left heel flat and toes pointed straight ahead
- Hold easy stretch 10 to 20 sec
- Do not bounce
- Repeat on other side
- Do not hold breath

Stretches calf

3

- Stand a little way from wall and place left hand on wall for support
- Standing straight, grasp top of left foot with right hand
- Pull heel toward buttock
- Hold 10 to 20 sec
- Repeat on other side

Stretches front of thigh (quadriceps)

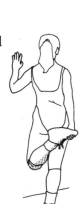

4

- Stand with feet pointed straight ahead, a little more than shoulder-width apart
- Bend right knee slightly and move left hip downward toward right knee
- Hold 10 to 15 sec
- Repeat on other side
- If necessary, hold on to something (chair, etc.) for balance

Stretches inner thigh, groin

5

- Move one leg forward until knee of forward leg is directly over ankle
- Place knee of other leg behind, resting on floor
- Lower front of hip directly downward to feel easy stretch
- Hold 10 to 20 sec
- Repeat on other side

Stretches front of hip and lower back; excellent stretch for lower back problems

6

- Sit on floor, legs straight out at sides
- Bend left leg in at knee
- Slowly bend forward from hips toward foot of straight leg until you feel slight stretch

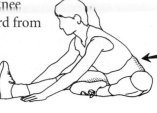

- Do not dip head forward at start of stretch
- Hold this developmental stretch 10 to 20 sec
- Repeat on other side
- Foot of straight leg upright, ankles and toes relaxed
- Use a towel if you cannot easily reach your feet

Stretches back of leg and lower back

7

- Lie on floor and bend right knee, foot flat
- Keep lower back flat on floor
- Lift left leg straight up from hip
- Lower leg down
- Hold for 10 to 20 sec
- Repeat on other side

Stretches hamstrings and calf

8

- Lie on left side and rest side of head in palm of left hand
- Hold top of right foot with right hand between toes and ankle joint
- Move front of right hip forward by contracting right butt (gluteus) muscles as you push right foot into right hand
- Keep body in straight line
- Hold easy stretch 10 to 15 sec
- Repeat on other side

Stretches front of thigh, hip, and ankles

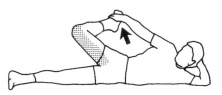

Do not hold your breath.
Stretch without comparing yourself to others.

BACK, SHOULDERS, ARMS, AND HANDS

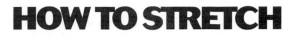

1

- Place hands shoulder-width apart on wall
- Bend knees; hips directly above feet
- Lower head between arms
- Hold stretch 10 to 15 sec

Stretches neck, shoulders, arms, and upper back

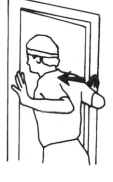

2

- Interlace fingers above head, palms upward
- Push arms slightly back and up
- Breathe easy
- Hold stretch 10 to 20 sec

Excellent for slumping shoulders; stretches arms, shoulders, and back

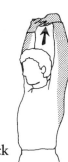

3

- Sit or stand with arms hanging loosely at sides
- Shrug shoulders up
- Hold 5 sec
- Breathe
- Then relax shoulders downward

Stretches shoulders, and neck

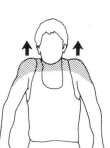

4

- Lean head sideways toward right shoulder
- With right hand gently pull left arm down and across, behind back
- Hold 10 sec
- Repeat on other side
- Relax

Stretches top of shoulders and neck

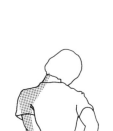

5

- Place hands shoulder height on either side of doorway
- Move upper body forward until you feel comfortable stretch
- Chest and head up, knees slightly bent
- Hold 15 sec
- Breathe easily

Stretches chest (pectorals) and inside of upper arms

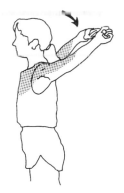

6

- Stand and hold towel behind you at both ends, hands far apart for free movement
- Straighten arms up and over head then down behind back
- Hold stretch at any place during movement
- Hold 10 to 15 sec
- Do not force a stretch

Stretches chest (pectorals) and inside of upper arms

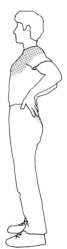

7

- Stand and place hands just above back of hips, elbows back
- Gently press forward
- Hold 10 to 15 sec
- Breathe easy
- Keep knees flexed
- Slightly lift breast bone upward as you hold stretch

Stretches chest (pectorals)

8

- Stand or sit and place right hand on left shoulder
- With left hand, pull right elbow across chest toward left shoulder and hold 10 to 15 sec
- Repeat on other side

Stretches side of shoulder and back of upper arm

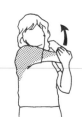

9

- Interlace fingers and turn palms out
- Extend arms in front at shoulder height
- Hold 10 to 20 sec, relax, and repeat

Stretches shoulder, middle back, arms, hands, fingers, wrist

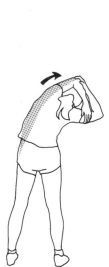

10

- Keep knees slightly flexed
- Stand or sit with arms overhead
- Hold elbow with hand of opposite arm
- Pull elbow behind head gently as you slowly lean to side until mild stretch is felt
- Hold 10 to 15 sec
- Repeat on other side

Stretches triceps, top of shoulders, waist

11

- Stand with hands on hips
- Gently twist torso at waist until stretch is felt
- Hold 10 to 15 sec
- Repeat on other side
- Keep knees slightly flexed

Stretches middle back

12

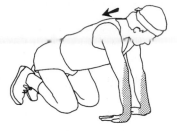

- Kneel on all fours with thumbs pointed out, fingers pointed toward knees
- Palms flat, gently lean back
- Hold 10 to 15 sec, relax, and repeat

Stretches forearms and wrists, which can be very tight areas of the body

13

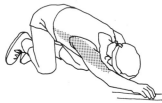

- Kneel with legs bent beneath you, rest forehead on left arm, and reach right arm forward
- Pull back at hips, pressing palms down
- Hold 10 to 20 sec
- Repeat on other side

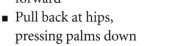

Stretches upper body (lats), shoulders, and arms

14

- Bend fingers at knuckles and squeeze for 10 sec
- Relax and repeat

Stretches hands and fingers

15

- Extend hands in front of you
- Separate and straighten fingers until stretching tension is felt
- Hold 10 sec, relax, and repeat

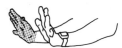

Stretches fingers and wrists

Listen to your body.
Enjoy stretching. It should feel good!

BACK AND NECK

HOW TO STRETCH

1

- Lie on floor and relax
- Bend knees, soles of feet together
- Lower knees out to sides
- Let gravity do the stretching
- Hold 10 to 30 sec

Stretches groin and hips

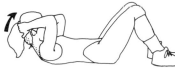

2

- Lie on floor, bend knees, keep feet flat
- Interlace fingers behind head at ear level
- Use arms to gently pull head forward, feel slight stretch
- Hold 4 to 5 sec, relax
- Repeat 3 times

Stretches neck and upper back

3

- Lie on floor, bend knees, feet flat
- Interlace fingers behind head at ear level
- Bring shoulder blades toward each other until tension is felt
- Hold 4 to 5 sec, relax and repeat

Stretches chest and helps the upper back relax

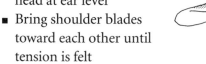

4

- Lie on floor, extend arms overhead, keep legs straight
- Reach arms and legs in opposite directions
- Stretch 5 sec, relax

Stretches shoulders, arms, hands, feet, and ankles

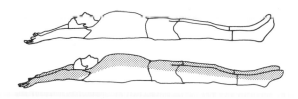

5

- Lie on floor, bend knees
- Extend one arm above head (palm up), other arm at side (palm down)
- Reach arms in opposite directions
- Hold 5 sec; both sides twice
- Keep lower back relaxed, flat on floor

Stretches arms and shoulders

6

- Lie on floor, legs straight
- Extend right arm above head (palms up), left arm by side, palm down
- Stretch diagonally
- Point toes of left foot as you extend right arm
- Stretch as far as is comfortable
- Hold 5 sec, then relax
- Reverse and stretch left arm and point toes of right foot

Stretches arms, legs, back

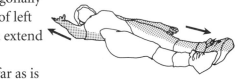

Relax your hands, jaw, feet, and shoulders

HOW TO STRETCH

BACK AND NECK

7

- Lie on floor, legs straight or with one leg bent (option)
- Gently pull right knee to chest
- Hold 10 to 30 sec, relax
- Repeat for other leg

Stretches lower back, hips, and hamstrings

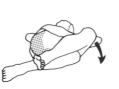

8

- Lie on floor, bend knees, cross left leg over right knee
- Interlace fingers behind head
- Use left leg to pull right leg toward floor until you feel mild stretch along side of hip and lower back
- Keep upper back, shoulders, and elbows flat on floor
- Stretch knee toward floor
- Hold 10-20 sec
- Repeat on other side

Stretches hips and legs

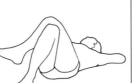

9

- Lie on floor, legs straight
- Bend left knee, extend left arm straight out from side
- Use right hand to pull knee across body
- Turn head toward left arm
- Keep shoulders flat on floor, feet and ankles relaxed
- Hold for 10 to 20 sec
- Stretch both sides

Stretches lower back and side of hip

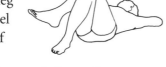

10

- Sit with fingers interlaced behind head, elbows straight out to sides, upper body aligned
- Pull shoulder blades together to create feeling of tension through upper back and shoulder blades
- Hold 5 sec, relax
- Repeat 1 to 3 times

Stretches shoulders and upper back

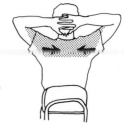

11

- Sit or stand with arms hanging loosely at sides
- Turn head to one side, then the other
- Hold for 5 sec, each side
- Repeat 1 to 3 times

Stretches side of neck

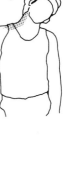

12

- Sit or stand with arms hanging loosely at sides
- Tilt head sideways, first one side then the other
- Hold for 5 sec
- Repeat 1-3 times

Stretches side of neck

13

- Sit or stand with arms hanging loosely at sides
- Gently tilt head forward to stretch back of neck
- Hold 5 sec
- Repeat 1-3 times

Stretches back of neck

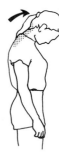

84

Learning proper technique will help you get the most out of weightlifting and will help prevent injuries.

REPS AND SETS   For each exercise in the Programs, we indicate *reps* and *sets*.

- *Rep* is short for repetition, or one complete movement (up and down or back and forth) of an exercise. Completion of a rep means you return to starting position.

- A *set* is a fixed number of reps.

HOW MUCH WEIGHT?   Use enough weight so you can complete the prescribed sets and reps fairly quickly, but the *last rep should feel difficult.* This will give your muscles the right amount of resistance (weight) to start making them stronger, but not so much that you injure yourself. As you make progress, and the last rep of the set starts feeling less strenuous, increase the weight, using the same principle.

PROPER POSITION   In a standing position, keep feet a little wider than shoulder-width apart and balanced fore and aft. Keep head and neck straight. Many lifting injuries are caused by twisting the head, neck, or trunk. When the spine is twisted, leverage is not as good and muscle injuries often occur. Always go through the full range of motion with each exercise. For bench position, see p. 8.

BREATHING   Inhale at the start of the lift, *momentarily* hold your breath during the most difficult part, and exhale as you finish. Breathe in and out through the nose *and* mouth. Do *not* hold your breath.

SAFETY

- Use collars on barbells. It's tempting to save time by leaving off collars, but the weights can slip off the end and cause injury.

- Use proper positions. Study the drawings.

- Don't jerk or twist when lifting. These movements increase stress and can cause injuries.

DAY OF REST   This simple principle is called *progressive resistance training. Always take a rest day in between weight training sessions.* A 24-hour rest period allows the muscles you've been working to adapt to the increased load. In weight training, you can easily stress or "overload" the muscle beyond the demands of previous activity. When this is followed by a rest period, the muscle(s) rebuild with greater strength.

NOTICE HOW YOU FEEL   On your day of rest, spend some time noticing the benefits of your training, a new and pleasant sensation of physical awareness. Almost immediately you'll feel firmer, improved muscle tone. You'll have more energy and a strong sense of how good it feels to move and be more active.

If you don't have that good feeling, you need to train harder. Increase the weights, add a few more reps to each set, or move ahead to the next level in the Programs. On the other hand, if you feel excessively sore or stiff, cut back some. You can expect a little discomfort as your muscles and joints adapt, but you should not feel pain.

1   DUMBBELL SWING

Most Large Muscle Groups

- Stand erect, feet 16 inches apart
- Hold dumbbell overhead with both hands
- Arms straight, squat until upper thighs are parallel to floor
- Raise up in semicircular motion with dumbbell at arms length until overhead
- Inhale up, exhale down
- Swing dumbbell through legs for better stretch

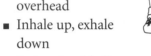

2   SEATED BARBELL TWIST

Obliques

- Sit at end of bench, feet flat on floor
- Place light barbell on shoulders
- Twist torso to right, then to left by twisting at waist only
- Do not move head from side to side
- Keep back straight, head up
- Inhale to right, exhale to left

(Can also be done standing; can also be done holding dumbbell next to chest)

3   BEND TO OPPOSITE FOOT

Obliques and Lower Back

- Stand erect, feet 16 inches apart
- Grasp dumbbell with left hand, palm in
- Bend until dumbbell nearly touches right foot
- Return to starting position
- Change dumbbell to right hand and repeat
- Inhale down, exhale up

4   HEEL-HIGH SIT-UP (ABDOMINAL CRUNCH)

Upper Abdominals

- Lie on floor, legs on top of bench (or against wall)
- Position body so thighs are at a 45° angle
- With hands behind head, crunch up as far as possible
- Return to starting position
- Do not swing body up and down but concentrate on abdominal muscles
- Exhale up, inhale down
- To make harder, hold light weight on chest

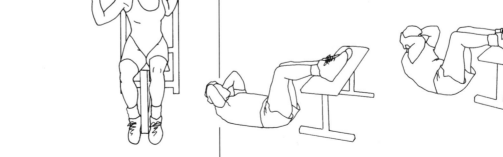

In Basic Program 5, put feet against wall

ABDOMINALS

5 BENT-KNEE ARMS-EXTENDED SIT-UP

Upper Abdominals

- Hook feet under strap of sit-up board
- Keep knees bent 45°
- Extend arms, elbows locked out
- Lie back until lower back touches and raise torso up and over until hands are above feet
- Exhale as you return to starting position

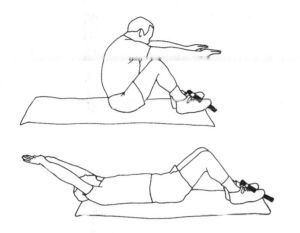

6 BENT-KNEE SIT-UP

Upper Abdominals

- Hook feet under strap of sit-up board
- Keep knees bent 45°
- Put hands behind head, chin on chest
- Lie back until lower back touches
- Return to starting position
- Inhale down, exhale up

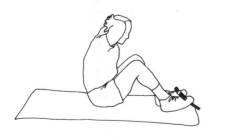

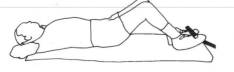

7 OVER-A-BENCH SIT-UP

Upper Abdominals

- Sit on bench
- Put feet under something to support body
- Keep knees slightly bent
- Bend back and down until just below parallel to floor
- Return to starting position
- Inhale down, exhale up

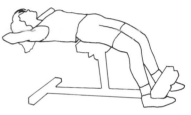

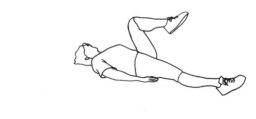

(To make harder, hold light weight on chest)

8 ALTERNATED LEG PULL-IN OFF FLOOR

Abdominals

- Lie on floor, legs straight out
- Bend knee as you lift right leg from hip
- Return to starting position
- Repeat with other leg
- Inhale up, exhale down

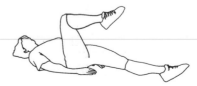

HOW TO LIFT

ABDOMINALS

9 LEG PULL-IN

Lower Abdominals

- Lie on floor with hands under buttocks, palms down, legs extended
- Bend knees, pulling upper thighs into midsection
- Return to starting position
- Concentrate on lower abdominals
- Inhale up, exhale down

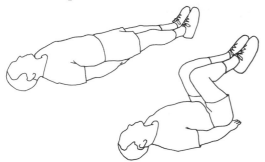

(To make harder, hold light dumbbell between feet)

10 FLAT BENCH BENT-KNEE LEG RAISE

Abdominals

- Lie on bench, legs hanging down
- Bend knees as you lift from hips
- Return to starting position
- Inhale up, exhale down

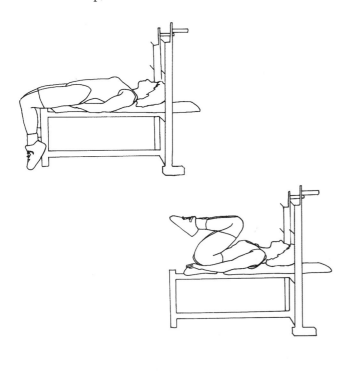

11 LEG PULL-IN OFF BENCH

Lower Abdominals

- Lie on flat bench with legs off end
- Hands under buttocks, palms down, legs out straight
- Bend knees, pulling upper thighs into midsection
- Return to starting position
- Concentrate on lower abdominals
- Inhale up, exhale down

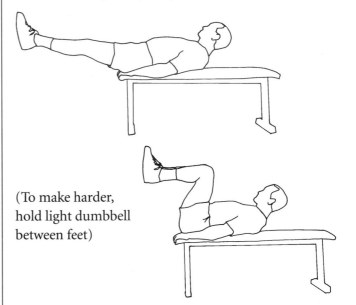

(To make harder, hold light dumbbell between feet)

12 ALTERNATED LEG RAISE OFF FLOOR

Abdominals

- Lie on floor
- Raise one leg, knee straight
- Return to floor
- Repeat with other leg
- Inhale up, exhale down

13 FLAT BENCH ALTERNATED LEG RAISE

Abdominals

- Lie on bench, legs straight out
- Raise one leg, knee straight
- Return to starting position
- Repeat with other leg
- Inhale up, exhale down

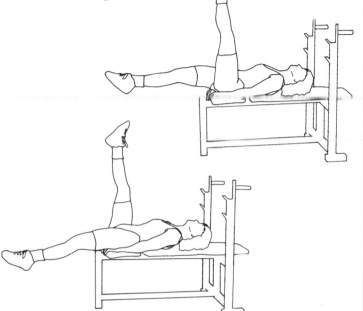

14 FLAT BENCH LEG RAISE

Abdominals

- Lie on bench, legs straight out
- Lift both legs straight up from hips
- Lower to starting position
- Inhale up, exhale down

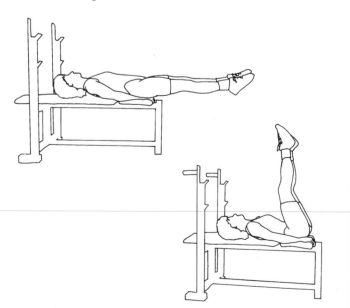

15 LYING SIDE LEG RAISE

Hips

- Lie on left side
- Tilt body slightly forward
- Raise right leg as far as possible
- Keep leg straight, do not bend at waist
- Return leg to starting position
- Lie on right side and repeat with left leg
- Inhale up, exhale down

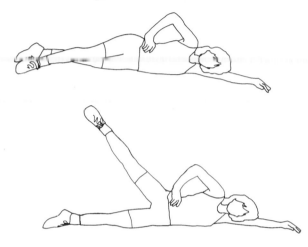

16 HIP ROLL

Obliques

- Lie on back
- Hold an object behind your head for support or place hands under buttocks, palms down
- Bend knees, feet firmly on floor
- Lower legs to right side until thigh touches floor
- Return to starting position, then repeat to left side
- Do all bending at waist
- Keep shoulders on floor
- Inhale to right, exhale to left

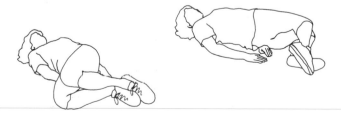

17   LYING LEG CROSSOVER

Hips and Obliques

- Lie on back and hold an object behind head with a wider-than-shoulder grip
- Keep shoulders on floor
- Swing right leg over left leg, as far to the side as possible until it is nearly as high as your head
- Keep leg close to floor
- Return to starting position, then repeat with left leg
- Keep knees locked, legs as straight as possible
- Inhale as you swing leg, exhale as you lower it

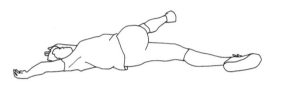

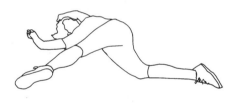

18   KNEELING SIDE LEG RAISE

Hips

- Kneel on bench, right leg hanging down
- Raise right leg straight out to side
- Lower to starting position
- Repeat on other side
- Inhale up, exhale down

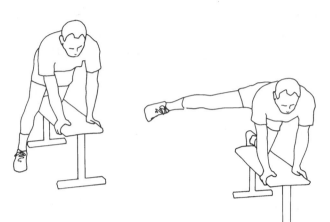

BACK

1 LYING BACK KICK

Lower Back

- Lie face down on floor; rest head on folded arms
- Lift left leg up from hip until you feel stretch
- Inhale up, exhale down
- Return to starting position
- Repeat on other side

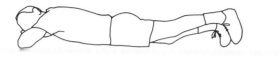

2 PELVIC RAISE

Lower Back

- Lie on floor, knees bent, feet flat on floor
- Keep arms straight on floor at side as you lift hips up
- Hold stretch and breathe
- Inhale up, exhale down
- Return to starting position

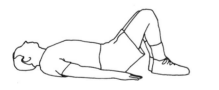
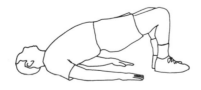

3 LAT STRETCH (DOOR KNOBS)

Upper Lats

- Hold doorknobs, stand straight, feet shoulder-width apart
- Bend knees to squat position
- Return to starting position
- Keep arms straight while squatting and returning to starting position
- Resist the movement with your upper back muscles

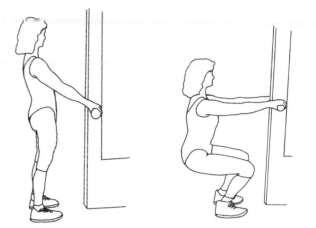

4 BARBELL GOOD MORNING

Lower Back and Abdominals

- Stand erect, feet 16 inches apart
- Place light barbell on shoulders
- Keep back straight, head up
- Bend forward until upper body is parallel to floor
- Return to starting position
- Keep knees locked
- Exhale down, inhale up

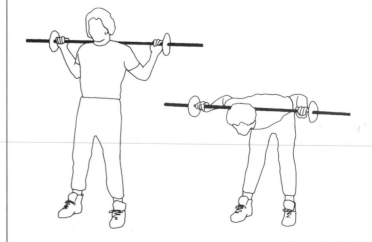

HOW TO LIFT

5 STIFF-LEGGED BARBELL DEAD LIFT

Obliques and Lower Back

- Place barbell on floor in front of you
- Hold feet 16 inches apart, bend, and grasp bar just to outside of legs
- Keep knees locked, back straight, head up
- Using only back muscles, stand erect with arms locked
- Lower weight to floor
- Inhale up, exhale down

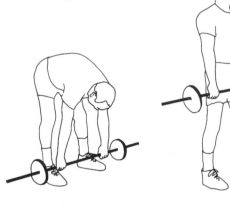

6 BARBELL SHOULDER SHRUG

Trapezius

- Hold barbell, palms down, hands 16 inches apart
- Keep feet about 16 inches apart
- Stand erect, bar hanging at arms' length
- Shrug shoulders up and rotate backwards in a circular motion from front to rear
- Inhale at beginning, exhale at end of repetition

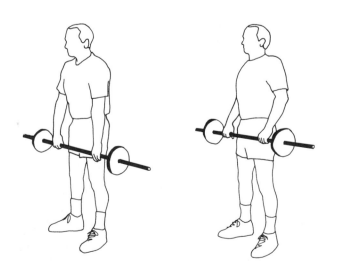

7 BENT-OVER DUMBBELL ROW

Lats

- Place dumbbell on floor in front of a waist-high bench
- Rest left forearm and forehead on bench
- Put right foot back about 36 inches, leg straight
- Bend left knee slightly
- Hold dumbbell with right hand
- Pull straight up to side of chest
- Lower to starting position
- Inhale up, exhale down
- Reverse position and repeat movement on left side

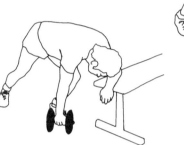

8 BENT-OVER ONE-ARM DUMBBELL ROW

Upper and Lower Lats

- Put right leg back, knee locked; bend left knee slightly
- Bend over and hold dumbbell with right hand, palm in, about 6 inches off the floor
- Pull dumbbell straight up to side of chest keeping arm close to side
- Return to starting position using same path
- Inhale up, exhale down
- Reverse position and repeat movement on left side

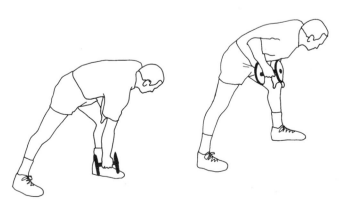

BACK

HOW TO LIFT

9 HEAD-SUPPORTED WIDE-GRIP BARBELL ROW

Upper Back and Upper Lats

- Place barbell on floor in front of you; feet 18 inches apart
- Place forehead on waist-high bench
- Bend over and hold bar in a wide grip
- Keep legs slightly bent and torso parallel to floor
- Pull bar straight up to chest; back straight
- Lower to starting position
- Inhale up, exhale down
- Do not let bar touch floor during exercise

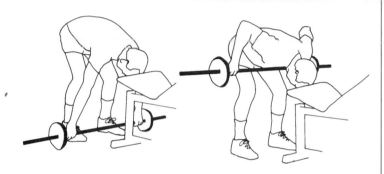

10 BENT-OVER WIDE-GRIP BARBELL ROW

Upper Back and Lats

- Place barbell on floor in front of you; feet 18 inches apart
- Bend over; hold bar with hands 6 to 8 inches wider than shoulders
- Keep legs slightly bent, torso parallel to floor
- Pull bar straight up to lower part of chest
- Keep head up, back straight
- Lower to starting position
- Inhale up, exhale down
- Do not let bar touch floor during exercise

11 HEAD-SUPPORTED TWO-ARM DUMBBELL ROW

Upper Back and Lats

- Feet close together; one dumbbell outside of each foot
- Bend forward and rest forehead on waist-high support
- Keep knees slightly bent
- Pull dumbbells straight up to sides of chest
- Lower to starting position
- Inhale up, exhale down
- Do not let dumbbells touch floor during exercise

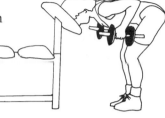
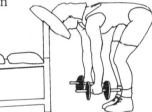

12 BENT-OVER TWO-ARM LONG BAR ROW

Upper Back and Lower Lats

- Place empty barbell bar in a corner or against something
- Put weights on upper end of bar
- Straddle bar; bend forward until torso is parallel to floor
- Keep knees slightly bent, back straight
- Hold bar just behind plates with both hands
- Pull bar straight up, elbows in, until plates touch chest
- Lower bar to starting position
- Inhale up, exhale down
- Do not let plates touch floor during exercise

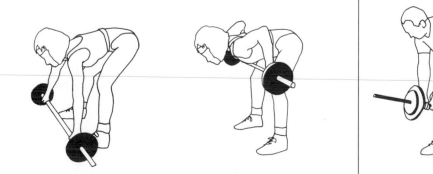

HOW TO LIFT

1 STANDING DUMBBELL CURL

Biceps

- Stand erect, feet 16 inches apart
- Hold dumbbells at arm's length, palms in
- Keep back straight, head up, hips and legs locked
- Begin curl with palms in until past thighs, then turn palms up for remainder of curl to shoulder
- Keep palms up while lowering until past thighs, then turn palms in
- Keep upper arms close to sides
- Concentrate on biceps while raising and lowering weights

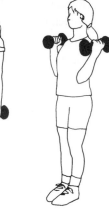

2 STANDING ALTERNATED DUMBBELL CURL

Biceps

- Stand erect, feet 16 inches apart
- Hold dumbbells at arm's length, palms in
- Keep back straight, head up, hips and legs locked
- Curl dumbbell in right hand with palm in until past thigh, then palm up for remainder of curl to shoulder
- Keep palms up while lowering until past thigh, then turn palms in
- Keep upper arms close to side
- Do a repetition with right arm, then curl left arm
- Inhale, up, exhale down

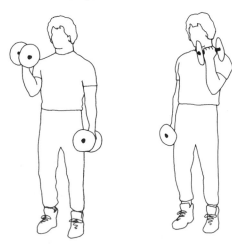

3 STANDING MEDIUM-GRIP BARBELL CURL

Biceps

- Stand erect, back straight, head up, feet 16 inches apart
- Hold barbell with both hands, palms up, 18 inches apart
- Start with bar at arm's length against upper thigh
- Curl bar up in semicircular motion until forearms touch biceps, upper arms close to sides
- Lower to starting position using same path
- Do not swing back and forth to help lift bar
- Inhale up, exhale down

4 STANDING CLOSE-GRIP BARBELL CURL

Biceps

- Stand erect, back straight, head up, feet 16 inches apart
- Hold barbell with both hands, palms up, 12 inches apart
- Start with bar at arm's length against upper thighs
- Curl bar up in semicircular motion until forearms touch biceps, upper arms close to sides
- Lower to starting position using same path
- Do not swing back and forth to help lift bar
- Inhale up, exhale down

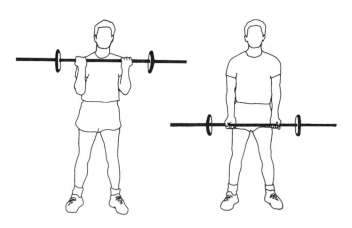

BICEPS

5 SEATED DUMBBELL CURL

Biceps

- Hold dumbbells
- Sit at end of bench, feet firmly on floor
- Keep back straight, head up
- Start with dumbbells at arm's length, palms in
- Begin curl with palms in until past thighs, then turn palms up for remainder of curl to shoulder height
- Keep palms up while lowering until past thighs, then turn palms in
- Keep upper arms close to side
- Concentrate on biceps while raising and lowering weights
- Inhale up, exhale down

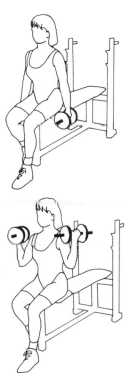

6 KNEELING CONCENTRATED DUMBBELL CURL

Biceps

- Hold dumbbell in right hand, palm up
- Kneel on left knee
- Right leg bent about 45°
- Left hand on hip
- Curl dumbbell up in semicircular motion to shoulder height
- Do not let upper arm rest against upper thigh
- Lower dumbbell to starting position using same path
- Inhale up, exhale down
- Reverse position and repeat movement with left arm

7 SEATED INCLINE DUMBBELL CURL

Biceps

- Hold dumbbells
- Sit on incline bench, dumbbells at arm's length, palms in
- Begin curl with palms in until past thighs, then turn palms up for remainder of curl to shoulder height
- Keep palms up while lowering until past upper thighs, then turn palms in
- Keep upper arms close to sides
- Inhale up, exhale down

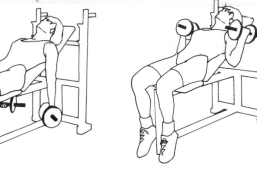

8 LYING INCLINE DUMBBELL CURL

Biceps

- Hold dumbbells
- Lie back on incline bench, dumbbells at arm's length, palms in
- Begin curl with palms in until past thighs, then turn palms up for remainder of curl to shoulder height
- Keep palms up while lowering until past upper thighs, then turn palms in
- Keep upper arms pointing down close to sides
- Inhale up, exhale down

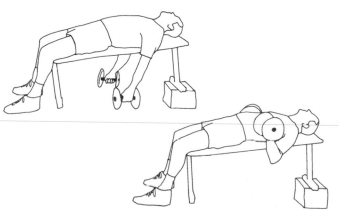

HOW TO LIFT

1 STANDING CALF STRETCH AGAINST WALL

Main Calf Muscles

- Stand on board facing wall, about 40 inches back from wall
- Lean forward with outstretched arms, hands against wall
- Keep back straight, head up, legs locked
- Rise up on toes as high as possible
- Do not let hips move backward or forward
- Hold momentarily, then return to starting position
- Inhale up, exhale down

2 TOE RAISE AGAINST WALL

Main Calf Muscles

- Stand facing wall about 40 inches back
- Lean forward and cross arms, hands on wall
- Keep back straight, head up, legs locked
- Rise up on toes as high as possible
- Do not let hips move backward or forward
- Hold momentarily, then return to starting position
- Inhale up, exhale down

3 STANDING ONE DUMBBELL TOE RAISE

Main Calf Muscles

- Stand with ball of left foot on board, 24 inches back from wall
- Hold dumbbell in left hand, hanging down at side, palm in, right hand on wall, right foot against left heel
- Keep back straight, head up, leg locked
- Rise up on toes as high as possible
- Do not let hips move backward or forward
- Hold momentarily, then return to starting position
- Inhale up, exhale down
- Reverse position and repeat movment with right leg

4 SEATED BARBELL TOE RAISE

Main Calf Muscles

- Sit on end of bench
- Hold barbell on upper thighs, 3 inches above knees
- Rise up on toes as high as possible
- Hold momentarily, then return to starting position
- Inhale up, exhale down

5 DONKEY TOE RAISE

Main Calf Muscles

- Place board on floor, 36 inches from bench
- Place balls of feet on board, legs together
- Bend forward and support upper body on bench
- Have training partner sit on your lower back with bulk of weight on your hips, legs straight
- Rise up on toes as high as possible
- Hold momentarily, then return to starting position
- Inhale up, exhale down

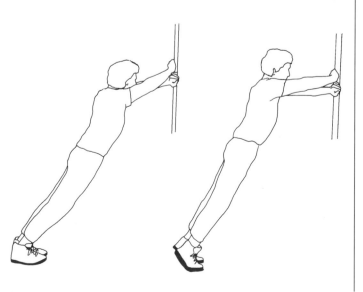

CHEST

1 INCLINE LATERAL

Pectorals

- Lie on incline bench
- Hold dumbbells at arm's length above shoulders
- Slowly lower so dumbbells are approximately even with chest, about 10 inches from sides of chest
- Keep elbows drawn downward and back in line with ears
- With forearms slightly out of vertical, press back to starting position using same arc
- Inhale at start, exhale at finish

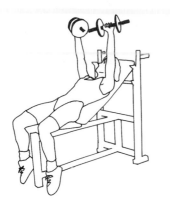

3 PUSHUPS

Pectorals and Triceps

- Kneel on floor, hands 12, 18, or 24 inches apart
- Place legs straight behind, back straight, head up
- Keep body rigid; lower yourself until chest touches floor
- Keep elbows in
- Pause at bottom, then press to starting position
- Inhale down, exhale up

In Super Circuit Training program, use close grip
In Chest Program, use wide grip
In On the Road Program, use close, medium, and wide grips

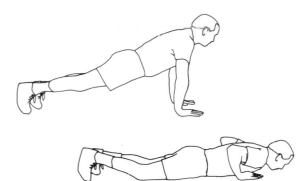

2 DECLINE LATERAL

Lower pectorals

- Lie on decline bench with two dumbbells together at arm's length above shoulders, palms in
- Slowly lower so dumbbells are even with chest, 10 inches from sides of chest
- Keep elbows drawn downward and back, in line with ears, forearms slightly out of vertical
- Press back to starting position using same arc
- Inhale at start, exhale at finish

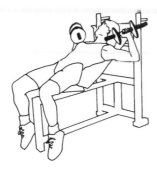

4 STRAIGHT-ARM DUMBBELL PULLOVER

Pectorals and Rib Cage

- Lie on bench, head at end, feet flat on floor
- Start with hands flat against inside plate of dumbbell at arm's length above chest
- Lower dumbbell in semicircular motion behind head as far as possible without pain
- Return dumbbell to starting position, elbows locked
- Inhale down, exhale up
- Breathe heavily, head on bench, chest high, hips on bench

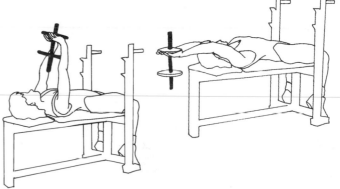

5   DIPS OFF SIDE OF DESK

Pectorals and Triceps

- Stand facing away from desk, hands holding on to edge, legs extended in front
- Bend arms and rest body weight on arms
- Hold stretch and breathe
- Return to standing position, exhale

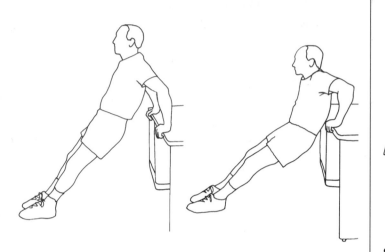

6   DIPS OFF BENCH

Pectorals and Triceps

- Stand facing away from bench, hands holding on to edge, knees slightly bent
- Bend arms and lower body to sitting position
- Hold stretch and breathe
- Return to starting position, exhale

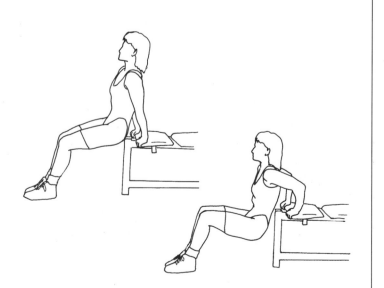

7   PUSHUP OFF SIDE OF DESK

Pectorals and Triceps

- Stand with feet together, hands on desk at arm's length
- Inhale and press forward, bending arms at elbows
- Keep legs straight, heels down
- Return to starting position, exhale

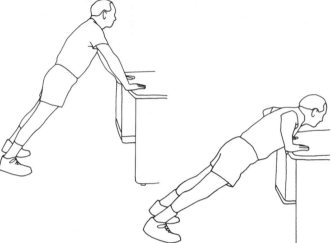

8   CHEST PRESS/DOOR JAMB

Pectorals and Triceps

- Stand with hands pressed against door jamb
- Keep feet shoulder-width apart
- Lean forward, bending arms at elbows, knees straight
- Return to starting position, exhale

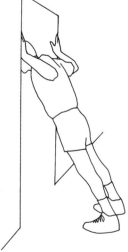

CHEST

HOW TO LIFT

9 FLOOR DUMBBELL FLY

Pectorals

- Lie on floor and hold a dumbbell in each hand at arm's length above shoulders, palms in
- Keeping arms straight, inhale and lower dumbbells in semicircular motion until weights are about even with side of chest but back slightly, nearly in line with ears
- Return weights to starting position using same path, exhale
- Breathe heavily, hold chest high, keep head down, and concentrate on pectorals

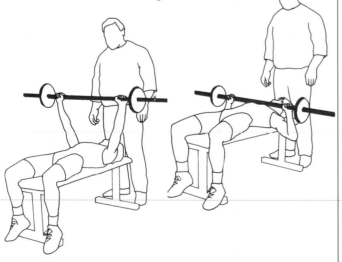

10 MEDIUM-GRIP BARBELL BENCH PRESS

Outer Pectorals

- Lie on bench
- Hold barbell 6 inches wider than shoulder width
- Lower bar to chest 1 inch below nipples
- Raise bar to arm's length, elbows out, chest high
- Keep head and hips on bench; do not arch back
- Lower weight with complete control, making definite pause at chest
- Inhale down, exhale up

11 BENT-ARM LATERAL

Outer Pectorals

- Lie on flat bench, dumbbells together at arm's length above shoulders, palms in
- Slowly lower so dumbbells are approximately even with chest, about 10 inches from each side of the chest
- Keep elbows drawn downwards, back in line with ears
- With forearms slightly out of vertical, press back to starting position using same arc
- Inhale at start, exhale at finish

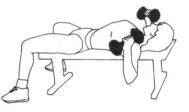

12 WIDE-GRIP INCLINE BARBELL BENCH PRESS

Outer and Upper Pectorals

- Lie on incline bench
- Use collar-to-collar grip
- Lower barbell to chest 3 inches above nipples
- Raise bar to arm's length, elbows back, hips on bench
- Lower weight with complete control, making definite pause at chest
- Keep head on bench, do not arch back too sharply
- Inhale down, exhale up

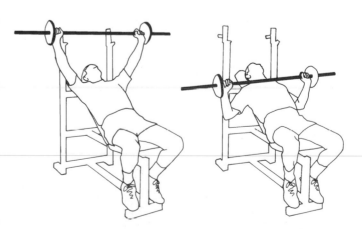

HOW TO LIFT

1 CLOSE-GRIP BARBELL UPRIGHT ROW

Front Deltoids and Trapezius

- Hold barbell, palms down, hands 6 to 8 inches apart
- Start with bar at arm's length
- Pull bar straight up until nearly under chin
- Keep elbows out, as high as ears; bar close to body
- Pause at top before lowering to starting position
- Inhale up, exhale down
- Concentrate on deltoids as you lower weight
- Can also be done with medium or wide grip

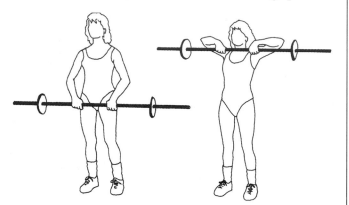

2 STANDING MEDIUM-GRIP FRONT BARBELL RAISE

Front Deltoids

- Stand with feet 16 inches apart, back straight, legs and hips locked
- Use shoulder-width grip; keep elbows locked
- Start with bar at arm's length against upper thighs
- Raise bar in semicircular motion until directly overhead
- Lower bar to starting position using same path
- Inhale up, exhale down
- Can also be done with close or wide grip

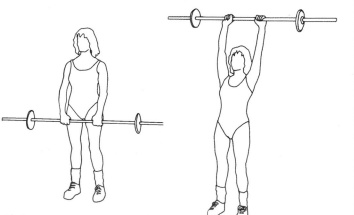

3 SEATED BACK-SUPPORTED SIDE LATERAL RAISE

Outer Deltoids

- Sit on bench, keep back against support
- Hold dumbbell in each hand, at arm's length, straight down
- Slowly raise weights in semicircular motion out to sides to a little above shoulder height
- Pause, then lower to starting position
- Keep arms as straight as possible
- Inhale up, exhale down

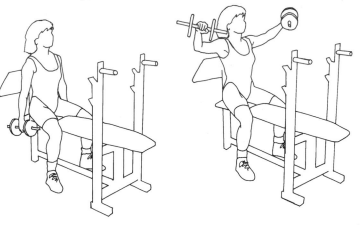

4 SEATED SIDE LATERAL RAISE

Front and Outer Deltoids

- Sit at end of bench, feet firmly on floor
- Hold dumbbells, palms in, arms straight down at sides
- Raise dumbbells in semicircular motion to a little above shoulder height
- Pause, then lower to starting position using same path
- Keep arms straight
- Inhale up, exhale down
- Can also be done standing

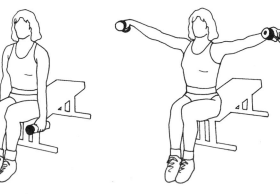

5 INCLINE REAR DELTOID RAISE

Rear Deltoids

- Lie face down on incline bench with dumbbell in each hand, palms facing each other
- Keep elbows locked and arms as straight as possible while raising dumbbells in semicircular motion to shoulder height, hands in line with ears
- Inhale up, exhale down

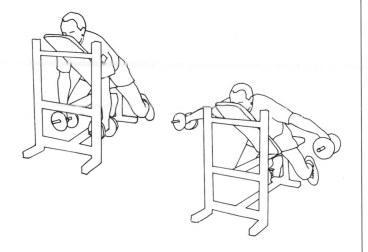

7 SEATED BARBELL MILITARY PRESS

Front and Outer Deltoids

- Sit at end of bench, feet firmly on floor
- Raise barbell to shoulders
- Keep chest high, back straight
- Press bar to arm's length overhead
- Use slow, steady motion, keeping tension on muscles
- Lower to starting position
- Inhale up, exhale down

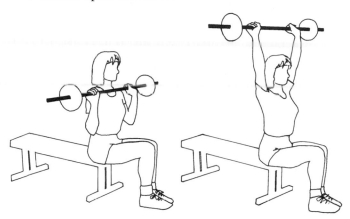

6 STANDING MILITARY PRESS

Front and Outer Deltoids

- Raise barbell to chest, hands shoulder-width apart
- Lock legs and hips solidly; hold chest high
- Keep elbows in, slightly under bar
- Press bar to arm's length overhead
- Lower to upper chest
- Be sure bar rests on chest and is not supported by arms between reps
- Inhale up, exhale down

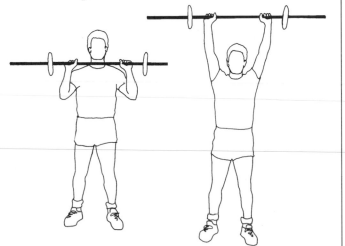

8 SEATED PALMS-OUT DUMBBELL PRESS

Front and Outer Deltoids

- Sit at end of bench, feet firmly on floor
- Raise dumbbells to shoulder height
- Keep elbows out, thumbs facing in
- Press dumbbells to arm's length overhead
- Lower weights to starting position
- Inhale at start of press, exhale at finish

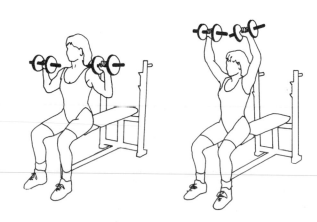

9 STANDING PALMS-IN ALTERNATED DUMBBELL PRESS

Front and Outer Deltoids

- Stand and raise dumbbells to shoulder height
- Lock legs and hips, elbows in, palms in
- Press dumbbell in right hand to arm's length overhead
- Lower to starting position and press other dumbbell up
- Keep body rigid; do not lean from side to side
- Do all work with shoulder and arms
- Inhale up, exhale down

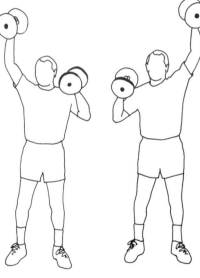

10 STANDING ONE-ARM DUMBBELL PRESS

Front and Outer Deltoids

- Stand and hold on to something with free hand
- Hold dumbbell with arm bent at shoulder height
- Lock legs and hips, elbows in, palms in
- Press dumbbell straight up to arm's length
- Return to starting position
- Repeat movement with other arm
- Inhale up, exhale down

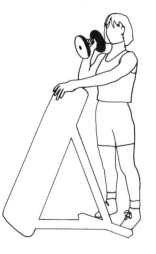

11 SEATED PALMS-IN ALTERNATED DUMBBELL PRESS

Front and Outer Deltoids

- Sit at end of bench, feet firmly on floor
- Raise dumbbells to shoulder height, palms and elbows in
- Press one dumbbell straight up to arm's length
- Lower to starting position and press other dumbbell up
- Keep body rigid; do not lean from side to side
- Do all work with shoulders and arms
- Inhale up, exhale down

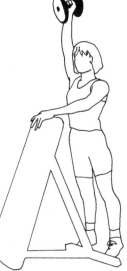

12 SEATED BARBELL PRESS BEHIND NECK

Front and Rear Deltoids

- Sit, feet about 16 inches apart, and place barbell on upper back
- Keep hands 4 to 6 inches wider than shoulders
- Press bar overhead to arm's length
- Lower to shoulders and pause
- Inhale up, exhale down

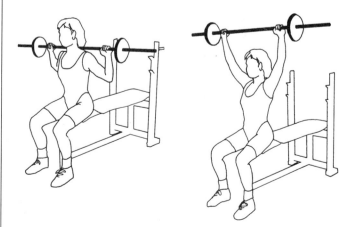

THIGHS

HOW TO LIFT

1 FREEHAND SQUAT TO BENCH

Upper Thighs

- Stand 16" in front of bench, arms crossed over chest
- Head up, back straight, feet 16 inches apart
- Squat until buttocks touch bench
- Keep tension on thighs; do not rest on bench
- Head stays up, back straight, knees slightly out
- Return to starting position
- Inhale down, exhale up

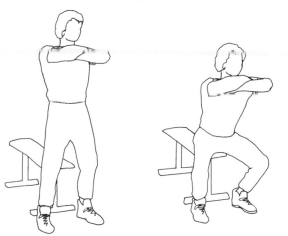

2 HEELS-ELEVATED MEDIUM-STANCE FREEHAND SQUAT

Upper Thighs

- Stand erect with arms crossed over chest, head up, back straight, feet 16 inches apart, heels on a board
- Inhale and squat until upper thighs are parallel to floor
- Keep head up, back straight, knees slightly out to sides
- Return to starting position as you exhale

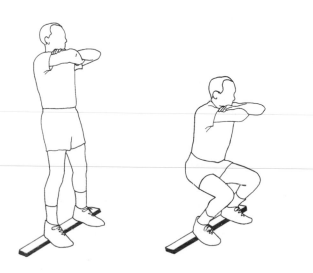

3 LEG EXTENSION

Lower Thighs

- Sit on bench with feet under lower foot pads as shown
- Have seat against back of knees
- Hold seat behind buttocks
- Point toes slightly down
- Raise weight up until legs are parallel to floor
- Return to starting position
- Inhale up, exhale down

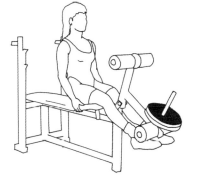

4 HEELS-ELEVATED MEDIUM-STANCE DUMBBELL SQUAT

Upper thighs

- Hold dumbbells at arm's length, palms in
- Head up, back straight, feet 16 inches apart, heels on a board
- Inhale and squat until thighs are parallel with floor
- Keep head up, back straight, knees slightly out to sides
- Return to starting position as you exhale

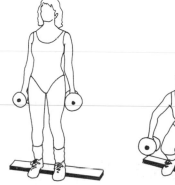

5   HEELS-ELEVATED MEDIUM-STANCE BARBELL SQUAT

Upper Thighs

- Stand erect, feet 16 inches apart, heels on a board
- Barbell rests on chest, on front deltoids and upper thorax
- Place hands on bar even with deltoids
- Keep upper arms above parallel to keep bar from sliding
- Squat until upper thighs are parallel to floor
- Head up, back straight, knees slightly out to sides
- Return to starting position
- Inhale down, exhale up

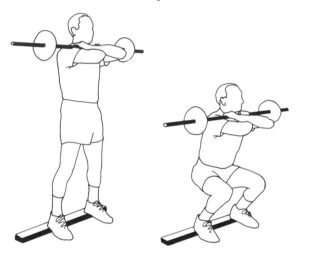

6   FLAT-FOOTED MEDIUM-STANCE BARBELL SQUAT

Thighs and Buttocks

- Place barbell on upper back; use comfortable hand grip
- Head up, back straight, feet 16 inches apart
- Inhale and squat until upper thighs are parallel to floor
- Keep head up, back straight, knees close together
- Return to starting position
- Inhale down, exhale up

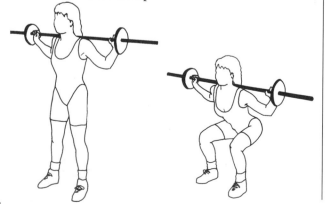

7   FREEHAND FRONT LUNGE

Thighs and Hamstrings

- Stand erect with hands on hips
- Back straight, head up, feet about 12 inches apart
- Step forward as far as possible with right leg until upper right thigh is almost parallel to floor
- Keep left leg as straight as possible
- Step back to starting position
- Inhale out, exhale back
- Repeat with left leg

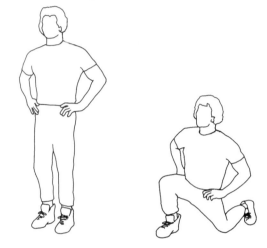

8   ALTERNATED FREEHAND FRONT LUNGE

Thighs and Hamstrings

- Stand erect with arms folded
- Back straight, head up, feet 12 inches apart
- Step forward as far as possible with right leg until upper right thigh is almost parallel to floor
- Keep left leg as straight as possible
- Step back to starting position
- Inhale out, exhale back

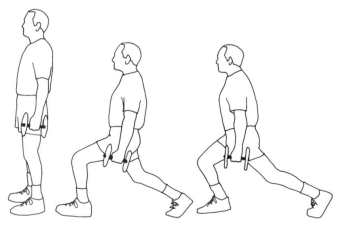

9 DUMBBELL FRONT LUNGE

Thighs and Hamstrings

- Hold dumbbells at arm's length, palms in
- Head up, back straight, feet 6 inches apart
- Step forward as far as possible with left leg until upper left thigh is almost parallel to floor
- Keep right leg as straight as possible
- Step back to starting position
- Inhale out, exhale back
- Repeat with right leg

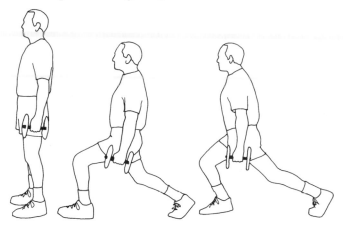

11 FREEHAND SQUAT

Upper Thighs

- Stand with arms crossed over chest
- Head up, back straight, feet 16 inches apart
- Squat until thighs are parallel to floor
- Head stays up, back straight, knees slightly out, hold
- Return to starting position
- Inhale down, exhale up

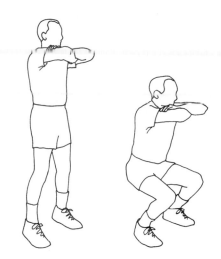

10 HEELS ELEVATED BARBELL HACK SQUAT

Inner and Lower Thighs

- Hold barbell behind you at arm's length
- Heels on a board about 30 inches apart
- Keep bar tucked against buttocks and upper thighs
- Palms facing back, hands as wide as hips, wrists up to lock bar solidly
- Head up, eyes up at 45° angle
- Squat until upper thighs are parallel to floor
- Return to starting position
- Inhale down, exhale up

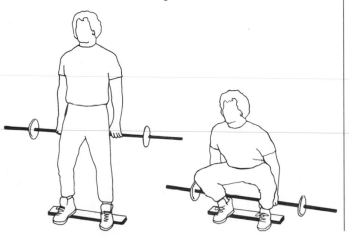

12 LEG CURL

Hamstrings

- Lie face down on bench
- Place heels under top foot pad
- Hold front of machine for support
- Curl legs up until calves touch leg biceps
- Return to starting position
- Inhale up, exhale down

HOW TO LIFT

1 TRICEPS PUSHUP/COUNTERTOP

Triceps

- Stand with feet 16 inches apart about 3 feet away from desk or countertop
- Place hands on edge and press forward until chest almost touches
- Keep back straight, head up, elbows out
- Inhale starting exercise, exhale at end

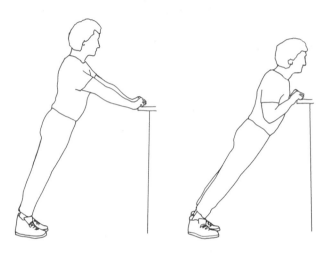

2 STANDING DUMBBELL TRICEPS CURL

Triceps

- Stand erect, head up, feet 16 inches apart
- Hold dumbbell with both hands; raise overhead to arm's length, upper arms close to head
- Top plates of dumbbell rest in palms, thumbs around handle
- Lower dumbbell in semicircular motion behind head until forearms touch biceps
- Return to starting position
- Inhale down, exhale up

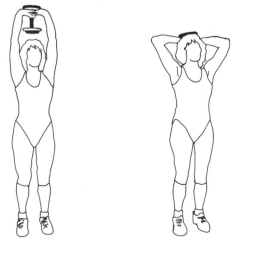

3 STANDING CLOSE-GRIP BARBELL TRICEPS CURL

Triceps

- Stand erect, head up, feet 16 inches apart
- Hold barbell with hands 6 inches apart, palms down
- Raise bar overhead to arm's length, upper arms close to sides of head
- Lower bar in semicircular motion behind head until forearms touch biceps
- Return to starting position
- Inhale down, exhale up

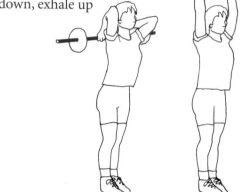

4 STANDING ONE-ARM DUMBBELL TRICEPS CURL

Triceps

- Stand erect, head up, feet 16 inches apart
- Hold dumbbell in right hand; raise overhead to arm's length, upper arm close to head
- Lower dumbbell in semicircular motion behind head until forearm touches biceps
- Return to starting position and repeat with left arm
- Inhale down, exhale up

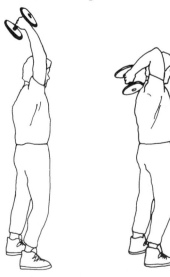

TRICEPS

5 SEATED CLOSE-GRIP BARBELL TRICEPS CURL

Triceps

- Sit at end of bench, feet on floor, back straight, head up
- Hold barbell with hands 6 inches apart, palms down
- Raise bar overhead to arms' length, upper arms close to head
- Lower bar behind head in semicircular motion until forearms touch biceps
- Return to starting position

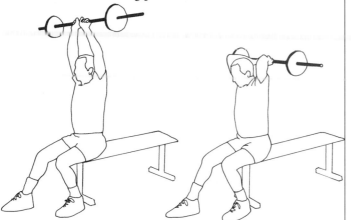

6 SEATED ONE-ARM DUMBBELL TRICEPS CURL

Triceps

- Sit at end of bench, feet on floor, back straight, head up
- Hold dumbbell in left hand; raise overhead to arm's length, upper arm close to head
- Lower dumbbell behind head in semicircular motion until forearm touches biceps
- Return to starting position and repeat with right arm
- Inhale down, exhale up

7 LYING ONE-ARM DUMBBELL TRICEPS CURL

Triceps

- Lie on floor
- Hold dumbbell in left hand at arm's length above shoulder
- Lower dumbbell in semicircular motion to side of head, bending arm at elbow, keeping upper arm vertical
- Return to starting position and repeat with right arm
- Inhale down, exhale up

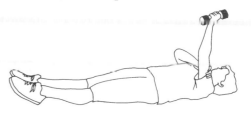
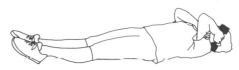

8 LYING CLOSE-GRIP BARBELL TRICEPS CURL TO CHIN

Triceps

- Lie on floor
- Hold barbell above shoulders at arm's length
- Inhale and lower barbell in semicircular motion, bending arms at elbows, keeping upper arms vertical
- Lower barbell to chin, until forearms touch biceps
- Press barbell back to starting position
- Inhale down, exhale up

9 LYING CLOSE-GRIP BARBELL TRICEPS CURL

Triceps

- Lie on flat bench
- Hold barbell above shoulders at arm's length
- Inhale and lower barbell in semicircular motion, bending arms at elbows, keeping upper arms vertical
- Lower barbell to forehead, until forearms touch biceps
- Press barbell back to starting position
- Inhale down, exhale up

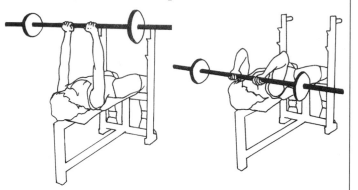

11 BENT-OVER TRICEPS EXTENSION

Triceps

- Stand with feet about 16 inches apart and bend over at waist
- Hold two dumbells at arm's length
- Bend arms at elbows
- Hold tension, then return to starting position

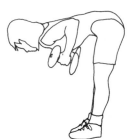
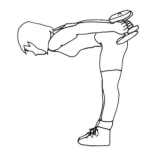

10 INCLINE CLOSE-GRIP BARBELL TRICEPS CURL

Triceps

- Lie back on incline bench
- Hold barbell with hands 6 inches apart, palms down
- Press bar overhead to arm's length
- Lower bar in semicircular motion behind head until forearms touch biceps, upper arms close to head
- Return to starting position
- Inhale down, exhale up

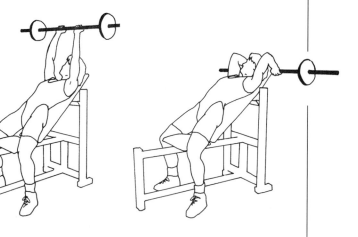

Doing something is better than doing nothing.

–Dr. Steven Blair, P.E.D.
Living with Exercise: Improving Your Health
Through Moderate Physical Activity

Who also says:

- Build physical activity into daily life
- Exercise needn't hurt
- Standing is better than sitting, moving is better than standing . . .
- Turn off the TV, get up off your fanny, go out the door
  and move around a bit

HISTORY OF HUMAN FITNESS

. . . the last two million years

NOMADIC LIFE

- Physical activity
- Gathering roots, seeds, fruits
- Chasing game
- Lots of movement
- 3–4 hours work daily
- Rest in between work periods
- Strength, health needed for survival

AGRICULTURAL REVOLUTION

- Plants cultivated
- Animals domesticated
- Tribes could remain in one place
- Life still very physical
- Plow, plant, harvest
- Lift, walk, carry
- Modern diseases unknown

INDUSTRIAL REVOLUTION

- Began 150 years ago
- Steam, internal combustion engines
- Move to cities
- Factory work
- Greatly increased food production, other products
- Standards of living rise
- Cities grow
- First evidence of high blood pressure, high cholesterol, etc.

ELECTRONIC REVOLUTION

- Personal computers, electronic wonders
- Much work becomes sedentary as machines do the heavy work
- *Stress*
- Air, water, other environmental problems
- TV, spectator sports, and entertainment create the couch potato
- Automobiles replace walking, buses, and streetcars
- Fast food, processed food, snack food, and junk food

. . . the last 25 years

THE '70s

- Publication of *Aerobics*, national bestseller: exercise improves health
- Marathon mania: Frank Shorter, Bill Rodgers heroes
- American College of Sports Medicine sets high fitness standards
- Millions of Americans start working out
- Huge fitness industry born

THE '80s

- High intensity workouts
- Triathlons
- Jane Fonda's "Go for the Burn"
- Hard-core training peaks
- Injuries mount
- People burn out
- Boredom

THE '90s

- "Fitness boom is a bust": only 10% of Americans work out
- A *lot* of information is available
- Lessons learned
- ACSM standards found to be unrealistic
- More balanced approach begins to unfold
- *Moderate* exercise discovered to provide high benefits
- Many activities besides running, cycling, swimming recognized as healthful (walking, gardening, housework, washing car, etc.)

THOUGHT

4 THE MAGNIFICENT HUMAN BODY

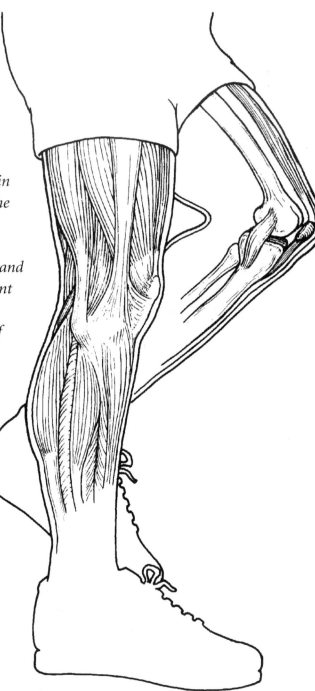

The amazing scheme of the human framework is to give support and protection while at the same time allowing great versatility of movement. The key to this versatility is the natural harmony and balance between the many and varied components of the framework and the ingenious way in which they are arranged.

The human skeleton is a structure which is flexible and yielding, yet firm enough to maintain the body in its characteristic upright position. The rigid elements are the more than 200 separate bones of which it is made up. Bones protect soft, vulnerable internal parts, particularly the brain and the spinal cord, and act as mediators of movement through a variety of intricate joints and the attachment of contractile muscles. Other types of muscle form an important part of such organs as the heart and digestive tract.

Other essential parts of the framework contribute to its vital plasticity. Connective tissue binds, packs and supports the internal organs. As cartilage it provides tough, friction-free surfaces at joints. As tendons and ligaments it creates links between muscles and bones, and as adipose tissue it forms an insulating and storage layer beneath the skin. The skin itself, the body's largest organ, is the tough, elastic outer fabric, resistant to water and the agents of disease . . . .

—Atlas of the Body
Rand McNally & Company

The human body is an incomparable instrument, a marvelous mechanism, breathtaking in its intricacy.

–Henry G. Bieler, M.D.
Food Is Your Best Medicine

The programs in this book, if followed, will cause changes in your body.

- *Stretching* moves your joints and muscles — you will be more flexible.
- *Lifting* strengthens your muscles, joints, tendons, and ligaments — you will look better.
- *Moving* improves the efficiency of your heart, lungs, and circulation — you will feel better.

Why will these changes occur? What's going on inside, under your skin? Here are a few facts about how your body works and the invisible changes that will take place internally as you become more fit with these programs.

THE WORKING SYSTEMS INSIDE YOU

The systems of the human body all work together in harmony so the body can move, twist, bend, walk, breathe, digest, heal itself, and perform innumerable other functions:

- The **heart, blood vessels,** and **lungs** provide oxygen and nutrients to the muscles and other cells.
- **Muscles** are the flesh or "meat" of the body. They control all movement in the body and make up 40 to 50% of its weight.
- **Bones** are the framework of the body. They make up the skeleton, providing internal structure and, in some areas, such as the head, external armor.
- **Joints** are where bones meet one another. Bones can't bend, but most joints can. To turn, bend, or twist any part of your body requires a joint.
- **Connective tissue,** including tendons and ligaments, connects muscles to bones, bones to bones, and anchors and cushions organs and other body parts.

The three systems of the body most affected by exercise are:

- **The Heart and Lungs**
- **The Muscles**
- **The Joints**

THE HEART

A person who is "big-hearted" is thought to be generous, romantic, and warm. Yet despite what the poets and storytellers tell us, the heart is basically a *muscle* — one that needs exercise to work well. The stronger it is, the better it works. A big heart may not make you more generous or romantic, but it will pump more blood around your body and deliver more oxygen and nutrients to the working muscles.

Your heart is the strongest muscle in your body and is about as big as your fist. It has a big job to do every day. Every minute of your life, even while you're at rest, the heart pumps five quarts of blood through your body. That's 2000 gallons every day, or enough to fill a tanker truck — travelling more than 60,000 miles through your blood vessels each day. In a year, your heart pumps enough blood to fill a supertanker.

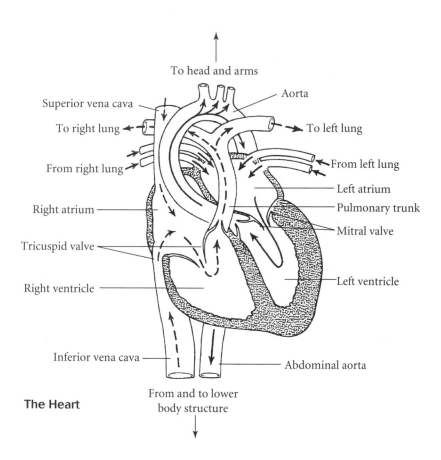

The Heart

WHAT HAPPENS TO YOUR HEART WHEN YOU EXERCISE?

When you start to exercise, various chemical and neurological signals tell the heart to pump faster and stronger. The heart responds like a rubber band. The more tension placed on the heart, the farther it stretches and the harder it snaps back, beating faster and pumping out more blood per beat.

BUILDING A STRONGER HEART

People don't generally think of the heart as a muscle; moreover, some don't understand that it can grow bigger and stronger just as other muscles can. All muscles respond to progressive resistance and endurance training, in which demands on the muscles are gradually increased.

You are undoubtedly familiar with progressive resistance training as practiced by bodybuilders: in lifting weights, the bodybuilder builds bigger and stronger muscles. That's easy to see. Well, the same principles apply to strengthening the heart (although the results are hidden from view). The right kind of training will cause the heart's muscle fibers to become thicker and stronger, resulting in a heart with greater muscle mass. The larger the heart muscle becomes, the more blood it pumps per beat.

Regular aerobic exercise produces a stronger and larger heart muscle that pumps blood more efficiently. And although exercising will cause your heart to beat faster, it will beat slower when you're at rest. And as you exercise regularly, other parts of your body become more efficient at extracting oxygen from the blood, further reducing the demand on your heart at rest.

After you achieve a certain comfortable pace while walking, running, swimming, cycling, or working, you may want to exercise at a higher intensity to place even greater demands on the heart muscle. Thus the heart will get *progressively* stronger and more efficient.

None of this happens overnight. It takes time. Remember, like all muscles, the heart takes time to grow. To strengthen the heart, you will need to exercise for an extended period of time (at least 20 minutes a day, 3 or more times a week) and you should start to feel significant changes after several weeks.

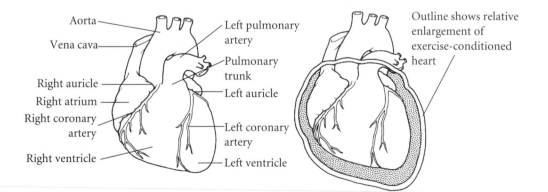

Normal Heart   **Athlete's Heart**

Normal heart compared to conditioned athlete's heart. A fit heart has:

1. *More muscle.* The heart muscle enlarges just like any other muscle with exercise.
2. *Slower rate.* A fit heart beats fewer times per minute at work and at rest.
3. *More power.* As the pulse rate goes down, the amount of blood pumped per beat goes up.
4. *Bigger arteries.* Arteries become larger than normal in diameter to allow for greater blood flow.

HEART RATE

To measure the effects of aerobic exercise on your heart, you need to know something about *heart rate*. As you begin exercising, your heart rate increases. During low-intensity exercise (that which you can sustain over a period of time), your elevated heart rate will level out at a constant rate (*steady state*). As you intensify the exercise, your heartbeat will increase proportionally. In other words, the faster you walk (or exercise), the faster your heart will beat.

Endurance athletes tend to develop big hearts with very slow resting heart rates. When Roger Bannister, the first person to break the 4-minute mile, began to train for his record attempt, his resting heart rate was in the low 70s. In peak shape (when he broke the record), his resting heart rate was down to 36 beats per minute. (Athletes generally take their resting heart rates when they first wake up in the morning, before getting out of bed.)

MAXIMUM HEART RATE

People have different maximum heart rates. Your rate and that of another person the same age might differ by as much as 10 to 20 beats per minute.

Maximum heart rate declines with age. Thus the maximum heart rate of a 60-year old will be much less than that of a 20-year old.

HOW HARD SHOULD YOU WORK YOUR HEART?

The best way to strengthen your heart is to exercise so that you raise your heart rate above a resting state and sustain it for a period of time. The best measure of the right intensity isn't how fast you walk, run, swim, or cycle, but how your heart, lungs, and muscles respond to exercise.

We've already discussed the fact that many (if not most) people will probably not want to follow a strict exercise prescription forever, but some may want to follow scientific guidelines.

Just like any medically prescribed treatment, cardiovascular exercise should be taken in proper doses if you want to get the most out of it and avoid any potential harmful effects. Many fitness leaders and medical personnel suggest the acronym FIT for an exercise prescription.

THE FIT EXERCISE PRESCRIPTION:

Frequency = number of days per week

Intensity = a measurement of your maximum heart rate

Time = the number of minutes you train per aerobic session

This is an effective prescription for aerobic fitness based on the principles of how often (*frequency*), how hard (*intensity*), and how long (*time*) you should exercise.

At an average resting rate of 72 beats per minute, your heart will beat over 100,000 times in 24 hours!

RULE OF THUMB: MAXIMUM HEART RATE

To get your maximum heart rate, subtract your age from 220.

THE AMERICAN COLLEGE OF SPORTS MEDICINE FITNESS GUIDELINES

Frequency: Exercise 3 to 5 times a week.

Intensity: Exercise at 60 to 90% of maximum heart rate.

Time: Exercise for 20 to 60 minutes each session.

When you begin, exercising *close* to your target heart rate will produce a cardiovascular training effect in your body. Don't worry about how fast you're walking or cycling. Just stay near the target heart rate. Here is how the calculation works:

Maximum heart rate = 220 minus your age

For example, if you are 45:   220 − 45 = 175

Your predicted maximum heart rate is 175 beats per minute.

TARGET HEART RATE

Your *target heart rate* is the rate at which you train. Here's the formula:

Lower level: Maximum heart rate (220 − age) × .60 = target heart rate

Upper level: Maximum heart rate (220 − age) × .90 = target heart rate

TARGET HEART RATE = THE RATE AT WHICH YOU TRAIN

Example for the same 45-year old:

Lower level = (220 − 45) × .60, or 175 × .60 = 105 beats per minute

Upper Level = (220 − 45) × .90, or 175 × .90 = 158 beats per minute

If you've been sedentary for a while, or are in an older age group, you should start out in the lower percentage range — 60%, *and sometimes lower.*

TALKING AND TRAINING

When exercising at 60%, you should be able to carry on a conversation with a training partner.

Pay attention to how you feel. If you feel uncomfortable at 60%, back off until you can keep up your activity for the prescribed time. Once again, this would apply especially if you're overweight, coming back from an injury, or haven't done much physical activity for years.

HOW TO TAKE YOUR HEART RATE

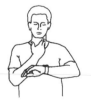

1. Pause during the exercise and take your pulse by placing index and middle fingers over either (a) your carotid artery on the side of the neck or (b) your wrist. Apply pressure lightly with your fingers.

2. Count for 10 seconds and use the **Ten-Second Heart Rate Conversion Table** *(next page)* to determine your heart rate in beats per minute.

3. Find the heart rate at which you are exercising by referring to the **Target Heart Rate (Percent of Maximum)** table *(next page)*. This will aid you in exercising in your training heart rate zone. Increase or decrease the intensity as needed to reach your target heart rate.

TARGET HEART RATE (PERCENT OF MAXIUM)*

AGE	60%	70%	75%	80%	85%	100%
under 20	126	147	158	168	179	210
20	120	140	150	160	170	200
25	117	137	146	156	166	195
30	114	133	142	152	162	190
35	111	130	139	148	157	185
40	108	126	135	144	153	180
45	105	123	131	140	149	175
50	102	119	127	136	145	170
55	99	116	124	132	140	165
60	96	112	120	128	136	160
65	93	109	116	124	132	155
70	90	105	112	120	128	150
75	87	102	109	116	123	145
80	84	98	105	112	119	140

NOTE

There are now several inexpensive wireless heart rate monitors available; a good one is made by Polar.

*Target heart rates must often be adjusted for individuals. Some people may have naturally high heart rates and be alarmed if their heart rates during training are higher than their calculated training zone. Others with naturally low heart rates may be frustrated by not being able to get their target heart rates high enough. Target heart rates may need to be adjusted to account for these differences.

TEN-SECOND HEART RATE

10-SECOND COUNT	BEATS PER MINUTE	10-SECOND COUNT	BEATS PER MINUTE	10-SECOND COUNT	BEATS PER MINUTE
8	48	17	102	26	156
9	54	18	108	27	162
10	60	19	114	28	168
11	66	20	120	29	174
12	72	21	126	30	180
13	78	22	132	31	186
14	84	23	138	32	192
15	90	24	144	33	198
16	96	25	150	34	204

PERCEIVED EXERTION METHOD

RULE OF THUMB: INTENSITY

Exercise slowly enough to be comfortable, but hard enough to get a training effect.

Recognizing that not everyone wants to do all the counting just described, the ASCM now has an alternative method of determining exercise intensity, called the *perceived exertion method.*

Here, you don't monitor your pulse during exercise. Instead, you make a subjective judgement as to how hard you feel you're working and try to keep it in the 60 to 90% (or the 50 to 80%) range. A good way to do this is to take your pulse enough times so you'll be able to make an educated guess from then on.

WHY DO SO MANY PEOPLE QUIT WORKING OUT?

Because they start out training too hard. Many may get so excited from early progress, they think "... if a little is good, a lot will be better." So they push hard, get exhausted or injured, and quit. *So take it easy.* Start slowly, especially if you haven't exercised for a while. Remember: the low end of this scale may be all you need to get and stay in good shape.

BLOOD PRESSURE

By now you know that your heartbeat is measured in beats-per-minute. Another measurement you should know about is that of *blood pressure.* When you have a physical, your doctor always checks your blood pressure. The ideal blood pressure is said to be 120/80. Just what is this measurement anyway?

In pumping blood around the whole body, the heart generates a lot of pressure. In a blood pressure test, your doctor measures two numbers:

- *Systolic* blood pressure = the higher number. This is the pressure in your blood vessels while the heart contracts and pumps blood.
- *Diastolic* blood pressure = the lower number. This is a measure of the reduced pressure in blood vessels when your heart is refilling between beats.

A healthy person sitting and reading this book might have systolic pressure of 120 millimeters (mm) of mercury and diastolic pressure of around 80 mm, commonly recorded as 120/80.

High blood pressure is said to start at 140/90 or higher. High blood pressure (also called *hypertension*) means extra work for your heart and blood vessels. Hypertension is second only to coronary artery disease as a major health problem. Research has shown that people who exercise tend to have a lower resting heart rate than most sedentary people. Thus, aerobic exercise can be one of the major factors in lowering blood pressure. *(See pp. 165–167 on high blood pressure.)*

THE LUNGS

So far, we've talked about cardiovascular training and its effect on the heart. Actually, your *lungs* are also part of the equation, since heart and lungs are so intimately linked.

THE HEART-LUNG TEAM

When you inhale, air enters the lungs. When you exhale, carbon dioxide exits the lungs. The lungs work in close partnership with the heart.

Your lungs work like bellows. They infuse the blood with oxygen when you inhale (air is 21% oxygen) and they expel carbon dioxide from the blood when you exhale. The oxygen and carbon dioxide are exchanged in the lungs' tiny air sacs, the *alveoli*. Here, they make direct contact with capillaries carrying blood. Oxygen-rich blood is pumped from the lungs to the left side of the heart. From there it is pumped through the body's largest artery, the aorta, to the rest of the body.

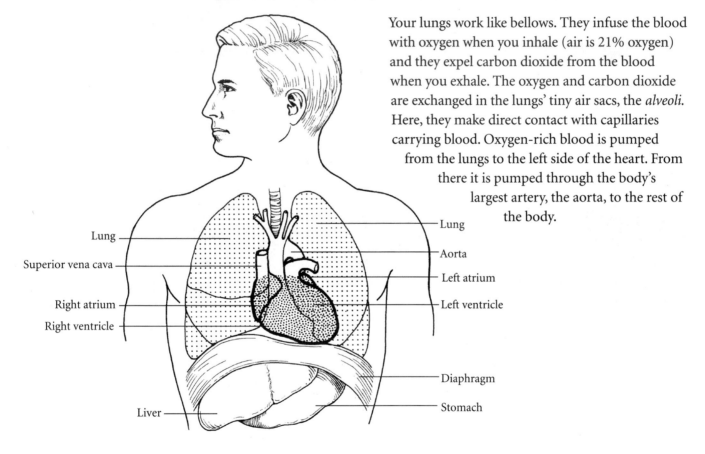

Lung

Superior vena cava

Right atrium

Right ventricle

Liver

Lung

Aorta

Left atrium

Left ventricle

Diaphragm

Stomach

THE EFFECT OF EXERCISE ON THE LUNGS

To begin with, the total area of the lungs is enormous — something like 40 times that of the outside surface area of the body.

Exercise increases the volume of the lungs slightly, and also causes their inner surface areas to increase. It is on these surface areas that the actual transfer of oxygen from air to red blood cells takes place.

THE MUSCLES

Muscles control all movement in the human body; they are the flesh or "meat" of the body.

JUST WHAT ARE THE MUSCLES?

Muscles are composed of cells; skeletal muscle cells are in the form of *fibers* — long, cylindrical cells bound together by a membrane. In most skeletal muscles, the fibers run the entire length of the muscle.

The fibers are bound together in bundles. To visualize this, think of a telephone wire (or bridge cable) with bundles of wire running along inside.

As we've said, having a sound heart (and lungs and blood vessels) is necessary for optimum health. But cardio-respiratory fitness is only one of the basics of a balanced fitness program. Having a good cardiovascular system doesn't necessarily mean you are in condition to go hiking with a full pack, or lift the occasional heavy box.

Biceps muscle

Fasciculus (bundle of muscle fibers)

Myofibril

Single muscle fiber

Section of biceps muscle (long head)

Column of myofibrils

The Architecture of Muscle

HOW DO THE MUSCLES WORK?

Muscles are cellular motors that move every part of your body. You can't walk, run, cycle, or lift this book without using your muscles. When a group of muscle cells (fibers) contracts, it shortens the entire muscle. The shortening pulls on the tendons which, in turn, move your bones. For example, when the quadriceps (front of thigh) contract, the lower leg is raised.

Muscles get nutrients from the bloodstream. To assure nourishment, each muscle has many blood vessels. Strong, well-developed muscles are filled with well-developed blood vessels.

As a muscle becomes stronger, the size of the cells increases, along with the number of blood vessels supplying the muscle. When you exercise, particularly against resistance, the diameter of the fibers thickens. This process is called *hypertrophy*. A bigger muscle is a stronger muscle and is more efficient.

121

JUST WHAT IS THE EFFECT OF EXERCISE ON THE MUSCLES?

Weight training exercise (called *progressive resistance* training) causes the muscles to get bigger and stronger. Further, increased muscular strength will give you more resistance to injury and will slow down the loss of muscle mass that nonexercising people experience as they get older. Aerobic exercise (*progressive endurance* training) increases blood flow, oxygen, and nutrients to the muscles being exercised.

Other benefits include improved appearance because your muscles will have *tone* — you'll look better and feel better. Your body will be more firm and you'll look younger. (As you get older, your body actually loses muscle — so-called fat-free weight — unless you exercise the muscles.)

THE OVERLOAD PRINCIPLE

Weight training is a part of just about every sport these days, from baseball to swimming to golf. Practically every serious and/or professional athlete knows about the *overload principle:*

> *For gains in strength or endurance, you must overload the muscle.*

But how does this apply to you? Even though you're not a pro, the same principle applies to anyone who lifts weights.

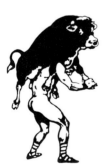

To "overload" a muscle simply means that you stress the muscle in intensity or duration *beyond the demands of previous activity.* This is then followed by a rest period in which the muscle will rebuild with greater strength and endurance. *(See p. 85 on the importance of a day of rest.)* The body does this by programming the cells to rebuild stronger so they can handle greater stress the next time. (It's one of the amazing automatic processes of the human body.) As your muscles adapt to the increased stress, you must overload them even more for further gains.

In 300 B.C., Milo of Croton demonstrated this principle — now called *progressive resistance training* — by hoisting a calf on his back every day until it became a full-grown bull.

HOW HARD SHOULD YOU WORK YOUR MUSCLES?

You should work hard enough to bring the overload principle into effect (if only slightly), but not hard enough to get exhausted or injured. In other words, *take it easy.* The surest way to make progress is to do so gradually. The key word is *progressive* resistance (or endurance) training.

THE JOINTS

The joints are the third part of our fitness equation. So far, we've talked about a healthy heart and strong muscles. Now we'll cover the important area of *flexibility*.

Flexibility is the ability to move joints through a range of motion — to bend, twist, and extend. Being able to use your muscles through their full range of motion makes physical work easier, helps improve athletic performance, and reduces chances of injury. Actions such as pulling weeds in the garden or throwing a softball require a fair degree of elasticity in some of your major muscle groups. Good flexibility is what allows you to use your full range of movement in a golf swing or to turn and look out the rear window of your car when driving.

THE ANATOMY OF A JOINT

Let's start with some definitions:

- A *joint* is a place where two bones meet.
- A *ligament* is a "belt" that fastens one bone to another.
- A *tendon* connects muscle to bone.
- *Cartilage* is a soft spongy material on the ends of most bones that cushions the contact between bones.

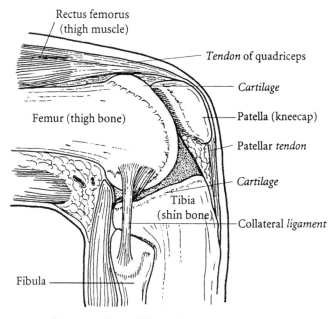

Rectus femorus (thigh muscle)

Tendon of quadriceps

Cartilage

Patella (kneecap)

Patellar *tendon*

Cartilage

Femur (thigh bone)

Tibia (shin bone)

Collateral *ligament*

Fibula

Cross-section of Knee Joint

DIFFERENT JOINTS HAVE DIFFERENT FUNCTIONS

Some joints, such as those between the bony plates of the skull, have grown together so tightly that they do not move at all. At the other extreme are the very flexible hip and shoulder joints — masterpieces of engineering that provide a phenomenal range of movement.

In a movable joint, ligaments and muscles hold the bones together. The ends of the bones are covered with cartilage which is smooth and slippery and protects the bones from injury. Around each joint is a fluid that lubricates the joint. Some joints have small sacs, called *bursae,* filled with fluid. The bursae act as shock absorbers. If they become injured, the condition is called *bursitis.*

The amount a particular joint can move is determined by the way the joint is built and the number and suppleness of the ligaments that hold the bones together. The ligament systems for your fingers, knees, and toes are similar: there are ligaments on each side of the joint that allow movement in one plane only. Your fingers and toes can only move in one plane, they cannot bend sideways. The wrist, elbow, and ankle have a wide range of motion: they can bend, flex, and rotate. Your arm can move in just about any direction at the shoulder joint. The hip joint allows your legs to move and your body to bend at the waist.

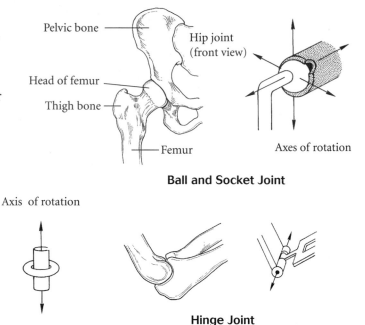

Ball and Socket Joint

Pelvic bone

Hip joint (front view)

Head of femur

Thigh bone

Femur

Axes of rotation

First two cervical vertebrae as seen from the back and slightly to the right side

Axis of rotation

Pivot Joint

Hinge Joint

WHAT IS FLEXIBILITY?

Flexibility refers to the range of motion in a joint or series of joints and is influenced by muscles, tendons, ligaments, bones, and bony structures.

Flexibility is determined by a number of factors. These include the level and type of activity being performed, with a fuller range of motion promoting greater flexibility and a limited range of motion inhibiting flexibility. Women are generally more flexible than men. Flexibility increases until the teen years and then decreases with age.

Temperature is also a factor — you're more flexible when it's warm and less so when it's cold. Flexibility is also highly specific to the joint being moved — you may be highly flexible in one joint, and have limited range of motion in another.

STATIC VS. DYNAMIC FLEXIBILITY

There are two basic types of flexibility:

- *Static flexibility* describes the range of motion about a joint without any reference to speed of movement. It is relatively easy to measure.
- *Dynamic flexibility* refers to the range of motion for a joint in action, and is much more difficult to measure.

It's obvious that static flexibility (how far you can bend, twist, or extend a joint while holding still) is not necessarily a good measure of the stiffness or looseness of that same joint when in action.

LACK OF FLEXIBILITY

Several conditions may occur to hamper joint flexibility:

- *Tendinitis* is an inflammation of the tendons. It can best be avoided by keeping the tendons supple.
- A *sprain* occurs when the ligaments in the joint are forced beyond their limits, and tear.
- A *dislocation* is when a joint is pulled out of its normal position.
- *Arthritis* may result from damage to a joint. It may be caused by wear and tear, injury, infection, or disease. *(See pp. 144–146 for a more complete description of arthritis.)*
- "*Creeping rigor mortis*" is our term for the accumulating stiffness that seems to come with aging. This stiffening is actually due more to inactivity than to aging. Without exercise, joints get stiffer and muscles become shorter and tighter.

THE ROLE OF STRETCHING

Just as aerobic exercise builds greater endurance (heart + lungs) and weight training is the key to greater strength (muscles), stretching is a way to maintain or increase flexibility (joints). Stretching is the simplest of these three activities. It doesn't require taking your pulse or counting minutes like aerobic activities, nor does it require equipment as does weight training. Further, it can be done anywhere, at any time.

Since range of motion is highly specific to each body part (shoulder, back, lower hip, etc.), a comprehensive stretching program that includes all body parts and follows the basic guidelines for flexibility development should be followed for best results.

The development and maintenance of good joint range of motion is important to good health and quality of life. Although body flexibility is partly determined by genetics, range of joint mobility can be increased and maintained through a regular stretching program and by working a muscle through a complete contraction and extension cycle.

SPORTS MEDICINE TITLES

- **Orthopedist** = treats muscular or skeletal injuries

- **Osteopath** = physician who uses manipulation and other techniques

- **Chiropractor** = spinal (and sometimes muscular) manipulation, realignment

- **Podiatrist** = treats foot, ankle problems

- **Physical therapist** = prescribes rehabilitation to restore function of body part

- **Sports nutritionist** = recommends diet to promote peak performance

- **Exercise physiologist** = designs individual exercise programs

5 FOOD

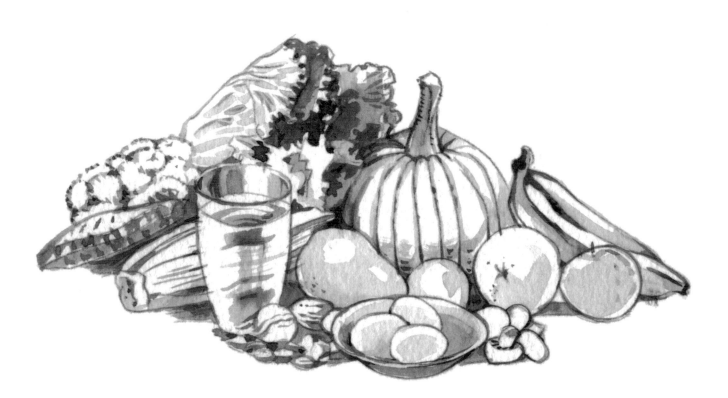

HEALTHY EATING

It is not the horse that draws the cart, but the oats.

–Russian proverb

There are currently over 2200 books in print in America concerning food, diet, and nutrition. (And this figure doesn't even include cookbooks.) Moreover thousands of magazine and newspaper articles are devoted to these topics annually. But since the food you eat, the diets you may contemplate, and the nutrition you receive play such important roles in good health, we'll briefly discuss some of the essentials. Hopefully, you'll keep these pointers in mind.

In 1985, the U. S. Department of Agriculture released its paper "Dietary Guidelines for Americans." Following are the guidelines, with the first two forming the framework for a good diet.

- Eat a variety of foods.
- Maintain desirable weight.
- Avoid too much fat, saturated fat, and cholesterol.
- Eat foods with adequate starch and fiber.
- Avoid too much sugar.
- Avoid too much sodium.
- If you drink alcoholic beverages, do so in moderation.

THE SURGEON GENERAL'S REPORT

In 1988, the first Surgeon General's Report on Nutrition and Health appeared, with its main conclusion being that "... overconsumption of certain dietary components is now a major concern for Americans. While many food factors are involved, chief among them is the disproportionate consumption of foods high in fats, often at the expense of foods high in complex carbohydrates and fiber that may be more conducive to health."

JULIA CHILD'S REPORT

If the Surgeon General's guidelines seem a bit stern, there's another approach you might want to keep in mind. In an interview in *Newsweek* in 1991, Julia Child said (and we paraphrase):

- One reason we overeat is because we eat too much processed food and not enough home cooking. Home cooking is satisfying.
- There's no bad food. There are just bad ways of using it.
- You can eat anything—but eat a small amount. You can eat a piece of beautiful chocolate cake with a butter-cream filling, but just eat a little piece.
- Dietitians and scientists put information in language people can't understand (grams, etc.) The public doesn't know what they're talking about. Thus, people don't understand the dietary guidelines.

SURGEON GENERAL'S DIETARY RECOMMENDATIONS ARE:

- Decrease consumption of fat (especially saturated fat) and cholesterol.
- Increase consumption of foods high in complex carbohydrates and fiber.
- Adjust caloric intake to achieve and maintain a desirable body weight.
- Consume alcohol in moderation, if at all.
- Reduce intake of sodium.

FAT

The best way to keep fat out of the arteries is to keep it out of the mouth.

–Bryant A. Stamford, Ph.D., and Porter Shimer
Fitness Without Exercise

WHAT IS FAT?

Dietary fat is one of the three major nutrients that provide energy to the body in the form of calories. The other two are protein and carbohydrates. The fat we eat may be obvious, such as butter on toast or whipped cream on a piece of cake. It's less obvious in foods such as nuts or milk, or when used as a recipe ingredient, such as oil or butter in a cracker or cookie recipe.

Dietary fat generally makes foods taste better by enhancing aroma, flavor, and texture. Since fat is digested more slowly than carbohydrate or protein, it remains in our stomachs longer and makes us feel full after we've eaten.

Fat has several essential functions: it is burned for energy by the muscles, especially during endurance exercise, it facilitates transmission of nerve and brain signals, it keeps the skin smooth, regulates body temperature, and cushions body organs.

WHAT IS CHOLESTEROL?

Cholesterol is a soft, waxy substance present in all parts of your body. It is a building block of the cells, vitamins, and hormones and is transported in the body through the bloodstream.

There are two sources:

1. Cholesterol made by your liver
2. Cholesterol you eat in animal products such as eggs, meat, dairy products, etc.

Studies have shown that a high intake of dietary cholesterol contributes to high serum cholesterol, which, in turn, increases risk of coronary heart disease.

GOOD CHOLESTEROL, BAD CHOLESTEROL

Cholesterol is transported through the bloodstream by lipoproteins, which are classified according to their density. There are two types:

- LDLs — the "bad guys" — *low-density lipoproteins,* which deposit cholesterol in coronary arteries
- HDLs — the "good guys" — *high-density lipoproteins,* the heroes that remove cholesterol from the artery walls and transport it back to the liver

"NO CHOLESTEROL"

For some years, some of the large food companies labelled cooking oils "No Cholesterol." The FDA felt this practice was misleading, as in fact all vegetable oils are free of cholesterol. The oils are still 100% fat, so the FDA instructed the food companies to cease such labelling. *Caveat emptor.*

GOOD FAT, BAD FAT

There are three types of fat, and they are of great interest to nutritionists and heart specialists because of their effect on cholesterol:

- *Saturated fats* are found in most animal products and some hydrogenated vegetable products and tropical oils. They are solid at room temperature. A diet rich in saturated fats interferes with the body's ability to clear excess cholesterol from the bloodstream. As layer after layer of deposits build up inside the blood vessels, like minerals building up inside a water pipe, the flow is restricted and oxygen and nutrients have a harder time reaching certain parts of the body.

- *Polyunsaturated fats* are found in such common oils as corn, safflower, sesame, soybean, and sunflower. Polyunsaturates help lower blood cholesterol by eliminating excess amounts. The drawback is that they reduce "good" HDL cholesterol, along with "bad" LDL cholesterol.

- *Monounsaturated fats* were previously thought to have a neutral effect on cholesterol. Researchers are now saying they appear to lower LDL levels without lowering HDL: a desirable effect. Canola, olive, almond, avocado, and peanut oil are in the monounsaturated category.

Here is a comparative chart of dietary fats.

HOW ABOUT SEMI-VEGETARIANISM?

Rather than being strictly vegetarian, try eating a diet of mostly vegetables, grains, legumes, fruit, and dairy products, with occasional servings of poultry, fish, or beef.

FATTY ACID COMPOSITION OF OILS AND FATS

% of Total Fatty Acids	Saturated	Monounsaturated	Polyunsaturated
Canola oil	6	62	32
Safflower oil	9	13	78
Sunflower oil	11	20	69
Corn oil	13	25	62
Olive oil	14	77	9
Soybean oil	15	24	61
Peanut oil	18	48	34
Sockeye salmon oil	20	55	25
Cottonseed oil	27	19	54
Lard	41	47	12
Palm oil	61	39	10
Beef tallow	52	44	4
Butterfat	66	30	4
Palm kernel oil	86	12	2
Coconut oil	92	6	2

HOW MUCH FAT DOES THE BODY NEED?

Some fat is absolutely necessary for bodily functions: for energy and to help store fat-soluble vitamins (A, D, E, K) in the body.

EIGHT SUGGESTIONS FOR CUTTING YOUR OIL BILL

1. Use half the amount of oil called for in a recipe. In most cases, it won't change the way the dish turns out.

2. Instead of pouring cooking oil into a pan, apply it with a brush or paper towel. All you need to do is add a thin coating to the pan to prevent sticking.

3. Watch your technique when sautéing or stir-frying. If you keep the heat high and stir constantly, you will need little or no oil to keep food from sticking.

4. "Sauté" with broth, juice, or water in place of oil.

5. Coat muffin tins or cookie sheets with a light film of canola oil, or use Teflon baking pans.

6. In recipes that call for a very flavorful fat like bacon fat, use one-quarter the amount. Make up the rest of the measure by using one-quarter unsaturated vegetable oil like canola, and for the remaining half, substitute water, vinegar, or stock.

7. Experiment with the darker, less refined oils such as walnut or grapeseed in place of the blander, highly refined ones. You can use less of them, since they do have a definite flavor.

8. Use liquid margarine instead of stick. It's less hydrogenated, and since you don't have to wait for it to melt on toast, you use less.

–Food and Nutrition magazine

You are what you eat.

–Anonymous

Fat Is Fattening   Americans today typically get 40 to 50% of their calories from fat. Of that, 15 to 20% is from saturated fat, 20 to 25% from fat that is unsaturated. For some years now, it has been obvious to medical professionals that this intake involves way too much fat. The Surgeon General, the American Heart Association, and the National Cancer Institute all recommend a maximum of 30%, with a proportion of 75 to 80% polyunsaturated, 10 to 15% monounsaturated, and 10% saturated.

FIBER

In the 1960s, British surgeon Dr. Denis Burkitt reported on population studies of rural Africans, whose diets consisted of foods with much higher fiber content than Europeans and Americans. The Africans showed a much lower rate of cancer of the large intestine, as well as significantly lower rates of constipation, diverticulitis, varicose veins, hemorrhoids, and coronary heart disease than Americans or Europeans.

Then, in the 1970s, Burkitt, along with colleagues, published a series of books and articles showing that a diet high in fiber would prevent a variety of digestive and other diseases. Within a few years, the high-fiber diet health fad was off and running.

WATCH OUT FOR UNHEALTHY "HEALTH" FOODS

For example, although the bran in bran muffins provides fiber, such muffins may also be loaded with sugar and fat (often hydrogenated oil). If a bakery muffin is heavy and sticky-surfaced, it may have as much fat and sugar as a doughnut.

RULE OF THUMB: FIBER

Include 25 to 35 grams of fiber (28 grams = 1 ounce) in your low-fat diet to reduce risk of diabetes, colon cancer, heart disease, and constipation.

FOOD	FIBER CONTENT
¼ cup raisins	2–3 grams
1 medium apple	3–4 grams
1 medium orange	3–4 grams
½ cup broccoli	2–3 grams
1 medium potato	2–3 grams
⅓ cup bran cereal (high fiber)	3–5 grams
1 cup whole wheat pasta	3–5 grams
⅔ cup lima beans	6–7 grams
¾ cup lentils	6–7 grams
⅔ cup kidney beans	6–7 grams

There have been articles, advertisements, even scores of cookbooks on the benefits of fiber and how to include more of it in one's diet. Clearly, in the 1990s, fiber has become well known for its beneficial effects, even for its life-saving possibilities.

But with all the data and the accompanying advertising hype a problem remains. You are left wondering how much fiber you should consume and what kind of products you should buy.

WHEAT VS. OATS

The truth is that there are two types of fiber, and they each do different things inside the body:

- *Insoluble fiber,* found in wheat, rye, fruits, and vegetables, cannot be digested. (A few generations ago, it was called roughage.) Insoluble fiber absorbs water and stays fairly intact as it passes through the digestive tract. It keeps foods moving from start to finish and helps prevent constipation and hemorrhoids. It is also thought to reduce the production of carcinogens in the intestines.

- *Soluble fiber,* found in oats, dried beans, peas, barley, and as pectin in most vegetables and some fruits, *does* break down, so it does not have the valuable bulking abilities of insoluble fiber. Before it breaks down, it forms a kind of gel as it absorbs water in the intestine. Because of this unusual characteristic, soluble fiber slows down the body's digestion of food, which means that glucose enters the blood stream at a slower rate, thus evening out sugar levels — good news for diabetics.

But the most significant advantage of soluble fiber seems to be its effect on cholesterol. Studies indicate that it consistently lowers LDL (bad) cholesterol levels, and has no significant effect on HDL (good) cholesterol.

FIBER TACTICS

Rather than lecture at length about the benefits of including more fiber in your diet, we simply point out that you should eat more whole grain breads, cereals, fresh fruits, and vegetables. We suggest you read the continuing stream of literature on the subject to determine what type and how much fiber to include in your diet.

We suggest that you don't make any radical changes right away. A significant increase in fiber can leave you feeling stuffed or bloated or running to the bathroom. Huge amounts of fiber can affect the body's ability to absorb important minerals such as calcium, iron, and copper. So take it slowly, learn as you go, and you should be able to find the right amount and type of fiber to improve your diet and your health.

DIETS

You go "on a diet." You go "off a diet." And by now you've probably learned, as millions have, that *diets don't work*. In fact, *Diets Don't Work* was the title of a best-selling book in the late 1980s. What the phrase actually means is:

- Radical diets don't work. Too much denial sets the stage for eventual failure.
- Diets alone don't work. There are other factors, foremost being *exercise,* that must be part of successful long-term weight control.
- Losing weight alone is not the key. On many diets, people are losing not only body fat, but lean, fat-free tissue (muscle).

WHY DIETS DON'T WORK

TIP: STEPPING ON THE SCALES

Don't weigh yourself more often than every week or two.

Here, in brief, are some reasons why diets (alone) don't work:

- Diets low in calories promote an initial large weight loss, but the loss is largely water.
- Too few calories, especially "starvation diets" (approximately 600 calories for women, 800 for men), causes the body to go into "starvation response." Metabolism — the body's calorie-burning mechanism — slows down significantly.
- Strict diets have their psychological drawbacks. Too much denial, too little fun in one of life's great pleasures — eating — set the stage for a pendulum swing in the other direction.
- This swing back and forth between losing weight, then gaining it back, is destructive. In fact, it's harder on people to lose weight and put it back on than it would be if they never lost weight in the first place.

"YO-YO DIETING"

Say you're overweight and you go on a low-calorie diet. To your satisfaction, you lose several pounds very quickly — the first week or so. The next week you don't lose as much — maybe a pound or so. By three or four weeks, you've reached a plateau and are losing little, if any, weight, even though you're still on the low-calorie diet.

As time passes, you develop cravings for forbidden foods. Finally you give in, have a few beers, or that piece of cake, and your earlier resolve is defeated. You're depressed and you abandon the diet.

Many people repeat this pattern over and over — it's called *weight cycling,* meaning repetitive cycles of weight loss and gain. Or *yo-yo dieting.* And the worst thing is, each time people put the weight back on again, they may end up a little fatter from the process, which means it will be even harder to lose the weight the next time they try.

A NEW TAKE ON THE SET POINT THEORY

The set point theory has been a popularly accepted supposition for some years now. The theory has been that your weight is held fairly constant by both biological and physiological influences and that as you eat less and start to lose weight, the body's metabolism will slow down unless you start to eat more once again. Depressing, isn't it?

Well, researchers at Cornell University recently came up with strong evidence that if you lose weight by reducing the total amount of *fat* in your diet, not carbohydrates, your metabolism will not slow down. Researchers think that metabolic rate may be related to carbohydrate consumption.

In ordinary weight-loss diets, calories are cut down with no thought as to whether they come from carbohydrates, protein, or fat. This Cornell research, then, is just one more factor pointing to the desirability of reducing fat, especially for those dieting. The results are encouraging news for those who thought that the set point theory meant they couldn't change.

DIETING VS. EXERCISE

CREEPING OBESITY

The main reason most people are overweight is lack of exercise, not overeating.

If you are going to try dieting, think about what exercise can do for you:

- Whereas dieting causes loss of both body fat and muscle, the right kind of exercise can preserve or even increase muscle. This fact is important since lean tissue (e.g., muscle) is metabolically active and burns calories.
- Whereas low-calorie diets reduce metabolic rate, exercise increases it. And not only do you burn calories while exercising, but your metabolic rate may stay higher for several hours *after* exercise. The longer and harder you exercise, the longer this effect persists. (Your body will burn more calories when you're at rest, even when you're asleep, due to higher metabolism.)
- Fat loss will occur more rapidly when exercise is added to the dieting program.

WON'T EXERCISE MAKE ME EAT MORE?

CREEPING LEANNESS

Adding 30 minutes per day of moderate exercise to your schedule can result in a loss of 25 pounds of fat in a year, even when food intake remains constant.

Many people believe that exercise will make you hungrier and therefore, you'll eat more and cancel out any weight loss — *not true!*

The fact is that most people who work out *moderately* (up to an hour a day) actually eat less than sedentary people. A lean person may eat more following increased activity, but the exercise will burn up the extra calories.

But the big difference (and the good news) is that if you have extra fat, you will react differently to exercise than those who are lean. Unless you exercise to excess, your appetite will generally not increase from the exercise. Why? Because when the body has excess stores of fat, the appetite is not stimulated by moderate exercise.

ACSM ON WEIGHT LOSS

The American College of Sports Medicine has published its position on weight loss programs. Here is a brief summary:

1. Prolonged fasting and extremely low-calorie diets can be medically dangerous. Along with rapid weight loss can come reductions in blood glucose, increased uric acid and ketone bodies, and reduction in blood volume and body fluids.

2. The goal in any weight reduction program is to lose body fat while retaining lean body mass (bone and muscle).

3. Cutting down on calories alone as a means of weight loss causes "moderate losses of water and lean body mass" — not a desirable effect. Additional drawbacks to the diet-only approach are reduced metabolism (your body burns less calories) and possible increase in LDL (the bad) cholesterol.

4. An exercise program involving ". . . dynamic exercise of large muscles . . ." will result in losing fat while retaining lean body mass.

5. A nutritionally sound diet with a reduction of 300 to 500 calories per day, together with an endurance exercise program, will promote fat loss and retention of lean body mass. You shouldn't lose any more than about two pounds a week.

6. Long-term weight loss involves a lifelong commitment, good eating habits, and frequent exercise. Crash diets and radical weight loss programs do not work.

A SIMPLER APPROACH

If all the foregoing sounds a little too scientific, here is what Douglas G. Swanson, a family doctor in Colorado Springs, Colorado, recommends to his patients in a newsletter. In fact, if you can remember these four tips, you'll be well on your way to a greatly improved diet:

1. *Avoid too much fat and eat what you want.* Dietary fat goes *directly* from your mouth to your waistline. Learn how to read labels.

2. Most people eat about 20 different dishes most of the time. Study these dishes and figure out how to lower the fat content without changing the taste significantly and keep eating them. That's it. That's all you have to do.

3. Your weight depends upon what you eat most of the time, not some of the time.

4. Occasionally eat whatever you want. If you feel deprived in your eating habits, you will not maintain them.

Tell me what you eat, and I will tell you what you are.

–J. A. Brillat-Savarin
La Physiologie du Goût, 1825

FINAL NOTE

Good health depends upon many things — heredity, environment, lifestyle, attitude, mental health, and exercise — in addition to diet. But nutritional knowledge, coupled with good eating habits based on variety and moderation, are the cornerstones in a foundation of good health.

RECOMMENDED READING

Safe Food: Eating Wisely in a Risky World by Michael F. Jacobson, Ph.D., Lisse Y. Lefferts and Anne Witte Garland © 1991. Living Planet Press, Venice, CA.

Jane Brody's Nutrition Book: A Lifetime Guide for Good Eating & Better Health & Weight Control by Jane Brody ©1987. Bantam Books, New York, NY.

Jane Brody's Good Food Book: Living the High Carbohydrate Way by Jane Brody ©1985. Bantam Books, New York, NY.

Nutrition, Weight Control, and Exercise by Frank I. Katch and William D. McArdle ©1988. Lea & Febiger, Malvern, PA.

6 PREGNANCY

EXERCISE DURING PREGNANCY

Pregnant women benefit from physical exercise in the same ways as do non-pregnant individuals, that is, with improved cardiovascular fitness, weight control, and mental well-being.

–The Physician and Sportsmedicine, July, 1991

Not many years ago, women who became pregnant were told to quit work and to "take it easy." These days, many health professionals advise pregnant women that regular exercise is good for both mother and child.

Before we go any further with this discussion we want to recommend an excellent book on the subject: *Essential Exercises For the Child-Bearing Year* by Elizabeth Noble, R.P.T. *(See p. 141 for details.)* But here, briefly, we'll give you some pointers on exercise during pregnancy.

PHYSICAL CHANGES IN THE MOTHER'S BODY DURING PREGNANCY

Several physical changes occur in a woman's body during pregnancy:

- Cardiac output and blood volume may increase by as much as 30 to 45%.
- Heart rate increases throughout pregnancy.
- Oxygen uptake (VO_2) increases throughout pregnancy and may be as much as 30% over nonpregnant values in late pregnancy.
- Estrogen and a hormone called relaxin are released in the body. These cause the body's ligaments to relax and the cartilage to soften. In addition, an increase of synovial fluid (the fluid that lubricates the joints) causes the pelvic joints to widen. These changes make birth easier, but they can lead to injuries from exercise during pregnancy if care is not taken.

EFFECTS OF EXERCISE ON THE BABY DURING PREGNANCY

As we know, everyone responds differently to exercise, and the same holds true for pregnant women. Factors such as age, weight, body composition, physical condition, and environmental conditions all influence your response to exercise.

There are some constants, however. Medical research shows three specific physiological areas of concern regarding the effects of exercise on the baby during pregnancy:

- *Blood flow to fetus.* Research has

shown that during moderate exercise, there may be a slight decrease in overall uterine blood flow. After exercise, blood flow quickly returns to normal.

- *Fetal temperature.* Exercise causes the body temperature to rise, and the temperature of the fetus rises as well.

- *Fetal metabolism.* Despite the fact that uterine blood flow decreases during exercise, glucose uptake by the uterus increases during exercise, and fetal metabolism does not seem to be affected. (This may mean that the fetus can take advantage of this energy mobilization and is not deprived of energy.)

FIRST CHECK WITH YOUR OBSTETRICIAN

Many physicians these days will recommend mild to moderate exercise for their pregnant patients. However, since everyone is different, there may be individual conditions that make exercise inadvisable. Thus, if you are pregnant and intend to exercise (or keep exercising), talk to your obstetrician first. Also, continue to consult your doctor about exercise as the pregnancy progresses.

GUIDELINES FOR EXERCISING DURING PREGNANCY

Keeping in mind these bodily changes during pregnancy, here are some general guidelines:

- Your core temperature should not exceed 101 degrees Fahrenheit. You should check your temperature rectally in the first trimester after a standard workout and keep the temperature under 101.

- Avoid saunas and hot tubs, and don't work out in hot, humid weather.

- Be careful exercising at high altitudes where air is thinner.

- The American College of Obstetricians and Gynecologists recommends keeping your heart rate below 140 beats per minute.

- Don't get anaerobic. In other words, don't get too far out of breath. A rule of thumb is that you should be able to carry on a conversation while exercising.

- Drink plenty of fluids before and after exercise. You are more likely to become dehydrated during pregnancy.

- Don't hold your breath when lifting weights or doing floor calisthenics.

- Avoid exercises like high-impact aerobics or fast changes in direction, since joints and ligaments are not as stable during pregnancy.

- Listen carefully to your body. If any unusual symptoms appear — pain, heart palpitations, shortness of breath, vaginal bleeding, etc. — stop exercising and consult your physician.

TYPE OF EXERCISE DURING PREGNANCY

Many pregnant women choose to continue their previous types of exercise during pregnancy, but have to reduce the duration and intensity.

- Swimming is the exercise of choice here. It is an excellent nonweight-bearing activity.

- Walking is also an excellent exercise.

- Some programs should be modified as pregnancy progresses; jogging or running must be cut back to less distance and eventually to walking.

- Cycling is a good nonweight-bearing activity. Riding a stationary bike is safer than riding on the road; for one thing, the change in center of gravity during pregnancy can affect balance.

- At present there is no specific data on the effect of weight training on pregnant women, but some medical experts feel that stronger muscles — developed by weight training — better enable a pregnant women to cope with the heavier body weight and altered center of gravity during pregancy. Stronger muscles also help the mother with the added chores of post-natal care, such as carrying the baby, washing diapers, etc. With your doctor's approval, weight training can be continued during pregnancy, provided the goal is strength maintenance and that you practice proper lifting and breathing techniques.

EXERCISES TO AVOID DURING PREGNANCY

Obviously, avoid sports such as rollerblading, waterskiing, horseback riding, or scuba diving and stick to low-impact aerobic movements. If it hurts while you're exercising, later in the evening or next day, don't do that exercise. Don't enter any competitive events while you're pregnant.

EXERCISE *AFTER* PREGNANCY

AFTER THE BABY IS BORN

There are two important rules to follow regarding exercise after pregnancy:

1. Listen to your body.
2. Listen to your doctor.

If you are sensitive enough to how your body feels, you will sense when it is all right to resume exercise. If you had a normal delivery, you can probably resume exercising as soon as you can do so without pain.

DR. KEGEL AND PELVIC MUSCLES

Arnold Kegel, professor of obstetrics and gynecology at the University of California at Los Angeles, did pioneering research in recent decades regarding the effects of exercise on

. . . the body undergoes hormonal and physical changes, which occur during the long months of pregnancy, but after delivery these changes are reversed within a matter of weeks. Labor and delivery thus signify an end and a beginning. The lengthy period of waiting and preparation is over, and so is the hard physical effort and excitement of the actual birth. But the greatest change and stress of the childbearing year occur after the arrival of the baby.

–Elizabeth Noble
Essential Exercises For the Child-bearing Year

improving female pelvic function. Many doctors and midwives now recommend that Kegel exercises be performed within a few days after the birth.

Kegel exercises are designed to strengthen the muscles of the pelvic floor. These muscles are extremely important because they support the contents of the pelvic cavity. (You can feel these muscles by stopping and starting the flow of urine.)

PELVIC FLOOR EXERCISES

The term *pelvic floor* refers to the muscles surrounding the vagina and urethra in front, and the anus to the rear.

1. Lie on your back or side (or front if you have had stitches). Draw up the pelvic floor and concentrate on tightening the sphincter surrounding the vagina and the urethra. Hold for 2 to 3 seconds, then relax, returning to a resting state. Do this 2 to 3 times, then rest for a few minutes.

2. While seated on the toilet, stop and start the flow of urine several times. As you continue to do this exercise over time, let smaller amounts of urine pass each time. This strengthens the muscles that support the bladder sphincter, and decreases incontinence after delivery and bladder infections.

3. Practice squeezing and releasing the anal sphincter. Strengthening the muscles that surround the rectum enables you to have more control over your bowels and tones the muscles of the entire pelvic floor.

A very complete chapter on the pelvic floor can be found in *Essential Exercises For the Child-bearing Year* (see p. 141).

AEROBIC EXERCISE

A woman who was physically active before and during pregnancy will respond to postpartum aerobic exercise more readily than a woman who did not previously exercise. If you are just now starting to exercise, take it *very* slowly.

For most women, the body begins functioning normally about two months after birth. As to the body's shape, exercise is the healthiest way to lose that weight. Once again, listen to your body, and listen to your doctor. Everyone is different. Some women will begin light exercising within a few weeks of birth, and others will require a month or more before it's comfortable to resume exercising.

Swimming and stationary cycling are ideal exercises because they are nonweight bearing. If you're a runner, walk before you (once again) run, avoid hard surfaces, and take it easy.

EXERCISE WHILE BREASTFEEDING

Women can exercise while they are breastfeeding, with certain precautions. The following suggestions are from Barbara Galloway, in *Galloway's Book on Running:*

- If milk quality or quantity decreases, stop aerobic exercise until the flow is normal. Also, increase fluid intake.
- Try to nurse just before exercising.
- You need extra calories: 400 to 500 more than when pregnant plus extra when exercising. (Don't use this as an excuse to overindulge, however. Get your extra calories from nutritious foods.)
- Use a bra with the greatest support.
- Take a nap with your baby whenever you can. Get extra sleep.

WEIGHT TRAINING AND STRETCHING

Both stretching and weight training are excellent activities for getting back in shape after pregnancy. See "Program Before the Program," pp. 15–18, for very gentle workout instructions that can apply to postpartum exercise.

CAUTIONS

As with exercise during pregnancy, most of the same cautions apply, except they become less important the farther you get away from the birthdate.

- Don't get dehydrated. Avoid exercising in high heat and high humidity. Stay out of saunas for a while. Drink lots of liquids.
- Keep your heartbeat down to 140, at least in the early postpartum stages.
- Stay away from high-impact sports, such as running or aerobics, until you get a green light from your physician at the postpartum examination. Remember, the ligaments and joints have softened to ease the rigors of birth and any jarring or sudden jumping movements can cause injury to loosened joints.
- Pay close attention to any discomfort or pain, such as uterine contractions, vaginal bleeding, nausea, dizziness, shortness of breath, pounding heartbeat, etc. Consult your physician.

RECOMMENDED READING

Essential Exercises For the Child-bearing Year by Elizabeth Noble © 1982. Houghton Mifflin, Boston, MA.

Shaping Up For a Healthy Pregnancy by Barbara B. Holstein © 1988. Human Kinetics Publishers, Champaign, IL.

Stretching for Pregnant Women. Wall chart. Stretching, Inc., Palmer Lake, CO.

Pre Natal and Post Natal Exercise Programs. Wall charts. California Gym Equipment Co., Los Angeles, CA.

Galloway's Book on Running by Jeff Galloway with Barbara Galloway © 1984. Shelter Publications, Bolinas, CA.

7 EXERCISE AND HEALTH

All parts of the body which have a function, if used in moderation and exercised in labours in which each is accustomed, become thereby healthy, well-developed, and age more slowly, but if unused and left idle, they become liable to disease, defective in growth, and age quickly.

–Hippocrates, 460–400 B.C.

Physical fitness is the basis for all other forms of excellence.

–John F. Kennedy

ABOUT EXERCISE AND HEALTH

This section briefly discusses some common medical concerns and how they relate to the exercise programs in this book. We are not specialists on any of these conditions, but we have researched each one of these fields in order to give you important new ideas. We've also listed the best literature available on each topic.

WHO SHOULD READ THIS SECTION?

People who have one or more of these conditions: You should be able to find some useful information to help you live in a healthful way with your condition.

People who do not have these problems: If you have a family history of any of these conditions or you are worried about any of them, you will find information here on ways to minimize your risks. Remember, an ounce of prevention . . .

THE EFFECTS OF EXERCISE

What's striking about recent research is that it shows that exercise has a beneficial effect on all these conditions. The more research that is done, the more evidence accumulates that exercise (at the proper time and in the proper amounts) will help. Exercise decreases the chances of contracting unhealthy medical conditions in the first place, helps you cope with them when they are already present, and delays progress of some of them. This applies from arthritis to back pain (the recommendation used to be "stay in bed") to osteoporosis to cancer, for which, until recently, exercise was not linked to any improvement in condition.

ARTHRITIS

(See Stretches for Arthritis, p. 147)

WHAT IS ARTHRITIS?

Arthritis is actually a symptom. It means "inflammation of the joints." To understand arthritis, it's important to know a little bit about the joints: joints allow the body to bend, flex, turn, and move. They provide flexibility, and they must also be strong. *(See. pp. 123–125)*

Joints make it possible for our bones to move while still supporting weight. With arthritis, we are not concerned with the muscles and tendons that enable the joints to move, nor with the tendons that provide joint stability. Rather, it is what goes on *inside* the joints that is of concern.

Inside the joints are two types of tissue: *cartilage,* which is slippery and allows the bones to slide smoothly when moved, and the *joint membrane,* which produces the fluid that feeds and cushions the cartilage.

The most common form of arthritis is what's called *osteoarthritis,* or (perhaps incorrectly) "wear and tear" arthritis. Of the 37 million Americans with arthritis, 17 million have this type. Here, the cartilage that covers and protects the ends of bones softens and may become pitted and frayed, or even wear completely away. The joints lose their cushioning, and pain results when the joints are moved. Another, less common form of arthritis is called *rheumatoid arthritis,* where the joint membranes become inflamed. Advanced rheumatoid arthritis is easy to recognize. Fingers and toes slant at odd angles. Joints are noticeably swollen. Doctors know the symptoms, but they don't know the cause of this crippling disease.

The best remedy for arthritis was commonly held to be rest. Wrong, says the Arthritis Foundation. Most doctors today prescribe exercise to combat pain and stiffening in arthritic joints. And, in the process, patients get the additional health benefits of cardiovascular training.

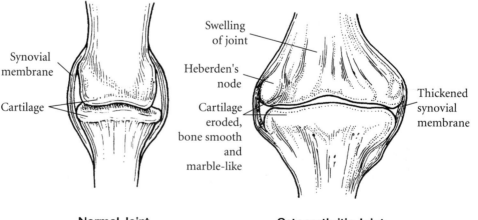

Normal Joint

Synovial membrane

Cartilage

Osteoarthritic Joint

Swelling of joint

Heberden's node

Cartilage eroded, bone smooth and marble-like

Thickened synovial membrane

IS OSTEOARTHRITIS REALLY CAUSED BY "WEAR AND TEAR"?

Many researchers speculate that it's not overuse that contributes to osteoarthritis, but rather *lack* of use. A sedentary lifestyle gradually reduces joint range-of-motion. This lack of movement is not the sole cause of arthritis, but there is increasing evidence that when joint and muscle groups are not moved, they atrophy. This resulting weakness makes joints even more unstable and everyday activities even more painful. The right type of exercise will keep you flexible and will lubricate the joints and strengthen the muscles, tendons, and ligaments that help support the joint structures.

Regular exercise helps keep joints flexible, helps build and preserve muscle strength, and helps protect joints from further stress.

–Arthritis Basic Facts Arthritis Foundation

WHAT HAPPENS WHEN YOU DON'T MOVE ENOUGH?

If you are mostly sedentary and do not exercise, your joints become stiff and your muscles smaller and weaker. People with a painful joint often keep it in a bent position because it feels better that way. But pretty soon, the joint can become locked, and loss of function and deformity can result.

WHAT TYPE OF EXERCISE IS BEST?

Running doesn't accelerate arthritis. Several studies on active people, including runners, show their chance of developing arthritis is the same as in sedentary people. Exercise is good for joints, and even the pounding from years of running doesn't increase arthritis risk. A recent study at the University of California Medical School, San Francisco, and Stanford University goes even further: Running doesn't even increase the rate of knee deterioration in runners who have arthritis.

Exercises emphasizing range of motion, strength, and endurance can lessen the effects of arthritis and may help prevent the onset of the disease. These are the three types of activity we recommend in all the programs in the book. Specifically:

■ *Range of motion* is best improved by stretching. If you have arthritis, try to move all affected joints through a full range of motion daily. *On p. 147 is a stretching program for arthritis.* To customize a stretching program, consult with your health professional and refer to the stretching index *(p. 206)* to find the stretches that are right for your individual condition.

■ *Strength* of joints and muscles can be improved by calisthenics or by doing *resistance exercises* with rubber bands. Strengthening the surrounding muscles will support and stabilize the arthritic joint. If your arthritis is not severe, you may even be able to do some light weight training, so long as you do not experience pain; but you need to be very careful here. Ask your doctor first. A doctor who believes in exercise for arthritis sufferers can help you choose the exercises best suited to your condition from the exercise index *(pp. 207–211)*.

■ *Endurance* activities, especially low-intensity *aerobic exercise,* can be of great benefit. High-impact activities, like running and aerobic dance, should generally be avoided, especially for those in the advanced stages of the disease, but vigorous cardiovascular training is encouraged when possible. Exercise bikes, rowing, and cross-country ski machines, as well as swimming and other water exercise (especially in warm water) all put less stress on your joints, since your weight is supported. Walking is another good activity, if it doesn't cause undue pain.

Resting is rusting.
Proverb

ISN'T REPEATED STRESS ON THE JOINTS HARMFUL?

Perhaps the most persistent myth about arthritis is that people should avoid physical activity because it will lead to further degeneration. The opposite is actually true. In a recent study of millworkers, seamstresses, and coal miners by Norton Hagler, M.D., professor of medicine at the University of North Carolina, the conclusion was: "There is no solid evidence that the repetitive use of joints causes damage to joints, muscles, or nerves."

CUSHION THE IMPACT, LIGHTEN THE LOAD

Although care should be taken to avoid high-impact activities, good equipment (such as well-cushioned running shoes and walking shoes) will aid in shock absorption. Weight loss is another beneficial measure. The less you weigh, the less stress on the joints when you move.

WARM UP AND STRETCH

It's especially important to start each exercise session with a good warmup to ease gently into exercise. Some gentle stretching and range-of-motion exercises both before and after the workout help prevent soreness and undue stiffness. Heat application (such as a hot shower, bath, Jacuzzi, or even topical applications such as Tiger Balm*) before and after exercise can feel great and improve range of motion.

PROGRESS MAY BE SLOW

A FINAL WORD

Exercise doesn't cause arthritis — but lack of it can.

Be patient. Slow progress is to be expected, especially if you've had arthritis for a long time. Expect some setbacks in any exercise program, but keep at it — the benefits will come. Remember, if weight training exercise produces pain that lasts longer than a few hours, cut back on either the repetitions performed or the weight. If cutting back doesn't help, choose a different activity that works the same joints and muscles, but does not cause pain. Also, exercise helps you *maintain* what strength and flexibility you already have, even if you don't improve that much.

RECOMMENDED READING

The Arthritis Helpbook by Kate Lorig and Dr. James Fries © 1990. Addison-Wesley Publishing Co., Reading, MA.

Arthritis — A Comprehensive Guide by Dr. James Fries © 1990. Addison-Wesley Publishing Co., Reading, MA.

The Arthritis Exercise Book by Gwen Ellert © 1990. Contemporary Books, Chicago, IL.

*Tiger Balm is a penetrating, heat-producing salve from China (in use for over 100 years). Write Pro Massage Co., P.O. Box 9220, Denver, CO 80209.

For information in general, contact The Arthritis Foundation, 1314 Spring St. N.W., Atlanta, GA 30309, 404-872-7100 or the local chapter closest to you (there are 71 chapters in the U.S.). The Foundation has 60 different pamphlets on various aspects of arthritis.

STRETCHES FOR ARTHRITIS

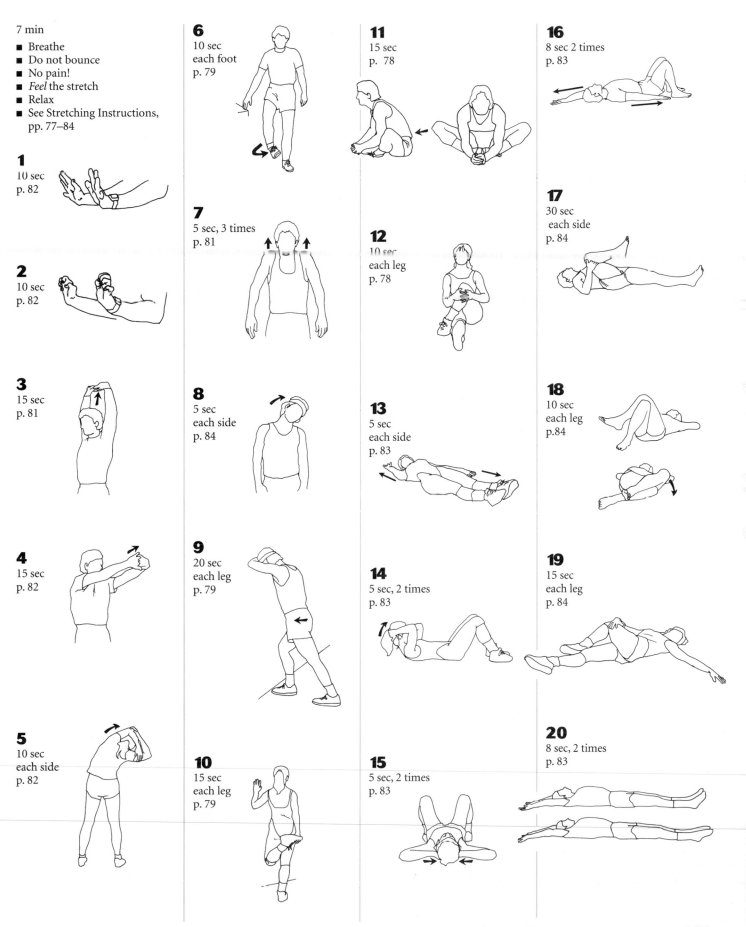

7 min
- Breathe
- Do not bounce
- No pain!
- *Feel* the stretch
- Relax
- See Stretching Instructions, pp. 77–84

1
10 sec
p. 82

2
10 sec
p. 82

3
15 sec
p. 81

4
15 sec
p. 82

5
10 sec
each side
p. 82

6
10 sec
each foot
p. 79

7
5 sec, 3 times
p. 81

8
5 sec
each side
p. 84

9
20 sec
each leg
p. 79

10
15 sec
each leg
p. 79

11
15 sec
p. 78

12
10 sec
each leg
p. 78

13
5 sec
each side
p. 83

14
5 sec, 2 times
p. 83

15
5 sec, 2 times
p. 83

16
8 sec 2 times
p. 83

17
30 sec
each side
p. 84

18
10 sec
each leg
p.84

19
15 sec
each leg
p. 84

20
8 sec, 2 times
p. 83

Photocopy this page and take it with you when you stretch.

BACK PAIN

Back pain, especially low back pain, is an epidemic in this country. By some estimates, as many as 80 to 90% of the population suffers from some type of lower-back ailment at one time or another. It's been estimated that back problems cost the nation as much as 10 billion dollars in medical care and lost work every year.

In some more vigorous societies, where people perform more physical labor and do not spend so long sitting or standing still, back problems are almost unknown. Back pain is primarily caused by our current life-styles, and fortunately this is an area over which we have some control.

ANATOMY OF THE BACK

The spinal column consists of vertebrae separated by discs that serve as shock absorbers. Together, the vertebrae provide a protective casing for the spinal cord and nerves that run up and down its channels. If these nerves or muscles surrounding the spinal column become irritated, compressed, or torn, problems and pain occur.

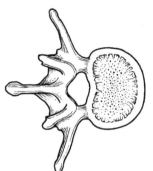

Single Vertebra
(top view)

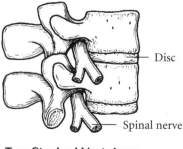

Disc

Spinal nerve

Two Stacked Vertebrae
(side view)

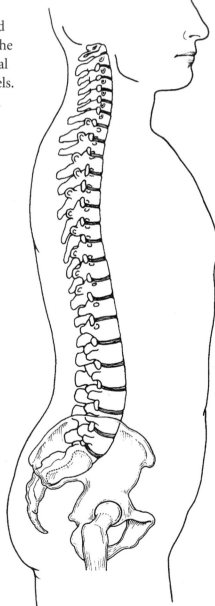

Spinal Column Showing the 24 Vertebrae

Back pain usually happens suddenly and can feel like a muscle spasm or a sudden pop. The feeling can be mild, or painful enough so that bed confinement is required.

PREVENTION IS THE KEY

The key to eliminating back pain is to prevent it before it occurs. Following are some important factors:

- Education about back care, proper lifting techniques
- Use of ergonomic workplace modifications (*see p. 163*).
- Weight control
- Exercise
- Stress reduction

WHAT MAKES FOR A STRONG SPINE?

Here is an important and often misunderstood fact: Primary support of the spine comes from the *muscles* and *ligaments* supporting the spine. Strength and stability of the spine do not come from the *bones* of the spine.

What's the significance of this? Many people feel that back problems are out of their control; it's a mysterious area and, further, they think they can't improve the strength of bones. But this isn't the case. You *do* have ways of getting better. Since the spine is held together by muscles and ligaments, you can improve a back problem by strengthening muscles and ligaments via exercise.

THE IMPORTANCE OF EXERCISE

"There's no evidence that bed rest works," says Paul B. Nutter, M.D., at Northwest Hospital in Seattle. He was quoted in a recent issue of *The Physician and Sportsmedicine* in an article on back pain entitled, "Out of the Bed and Into the Gym." Not only is bed rest ineffective, the article reports, but many experts today feel it leads to deterioration of the muscular and cardiovascular systems. Several studies were cited that ". . . overwhelmingly favor activity for back pain."

WHAT AREAS TO EXERCISE

For a strong back, two main areas need to be strengthened:

- Lower back muscles
- Abdominal muscles

Strengthening the muscles and ligaments of the lower back will give the spine the strong support it needs for injury-free functioning. Strong abdominal muscles reduce the stress on the lower back by taking on their share of the load.

Of patients complaining of back pain, only about 1% need surgery . . . that means, obviously, that the great majority should be treated nonsurgically. Exercise is an integral part of both the nonsurgical treatment and the postsurgical treatment.

–Stanley Herring, M.D.
Puget Sound Sports Physicians
The Physician and Sportsmedicine

STRETCHING

Exercises that stretch the lower back and leg muscles are of great benefit. By reducing or eliminating stiffness in these muscles, stretching can relieve much of the tightness that contributes to a bad back. Flexible and relaxed muscles are better able to handle the dynamic movements to which we subject our backs.

SITTING VS. ACTIVITY

Many back problems come from people sitting too much and not using their abdominal and back muscles. The sedentary life takes its toll, while vigorous activity promotes better abdominal-back functioning.

THE ABDOMINAL-BACK UNIT

Think of your abdominals and back as a unit. Develop these muscles to increase total body fitness and to fend off back problems. Pay more attention to stretching and strengthening the back and abdominals and you will have a fit midsection.

STRESS AND BACK PAIN

Dr. John Sarno, a professor of clinical rehabilitation at the New York University School of Medicine, has a unique theory on back pain. After treating thousands of patients for back pain over a 17-year period, Arno claims that the overwhelming majority of back-pain sufferers have been misdiagnosed — that doctors have been treating the *symptoms* rather than the underlying *cause*. Back pain, he claims, is almost always stress-related. He has observed that many back-pain sufferers are perfectionists — competitive-type people — and that the stress they experience reduces blood flow to various tissues in the back region. In his book, *Mind Over Back Pain (see below),* he outlines a mental therapy that is said to have cured thousands of people's back problems.

RECOMMENDED READING

Maggie's Back Book by Maggie Lettvin © 1976. Houghton Mifflin, Boston, MA.

The Goodbye Back Pain Handbook by J. A. Peterson and J. Wheeler © 1988. Masters Press, Grand Rapids, MI.

Mind Over Back Pain by John Sarno, M.D. © 1987. Berkley Publishers, New York, NY.

Healing Back Pain by John Sarno, M.D. © 1991. Warner Books, New York, NY.

Stretching by Bob and Jean Anderson © 1980. Shelter Publications, Bolinas, CA.

Back Designs — catalog of chairs, seat cushions, tools for people with back problems. 614 Grand Avenue, Oakland, CA., 415-451-6600

BACK PAIN

Stretch every day.
Lift OR Move on alternate days.
This program will take 20–30 minutes.

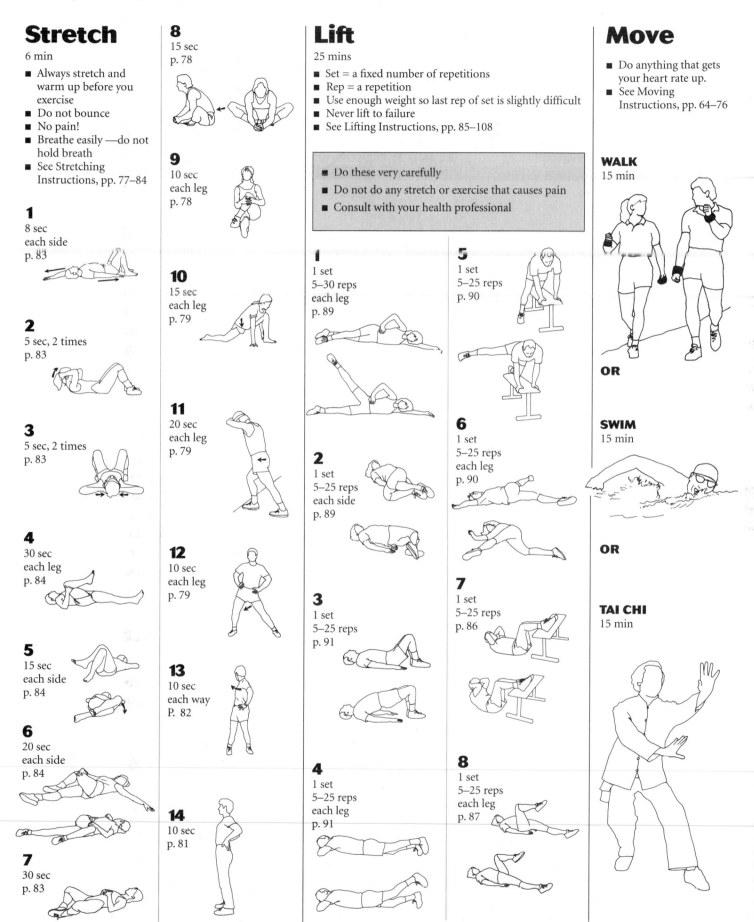

Stretch
6 min

- Always stretch and warm up before you exercise
- Do not bounce
- No pain!
- Breathe easily —do not hold breath
- See Stretching Instructions, pp. 77–84

1
8 sec
each side
p. 83

2
5 sec, 2 times
p. 83

3
5 sec, 2 times
p. 83

4
30 sec
each leg
p. 84

5
15 sec
each side
p. 84

6
20 sec
each side
p. 84

7
30 sec
p. 83

8
15 sec
p. 78

9
10 sec
each leg
p. 78

10
15 sec
each leg
p. 79

11
20 sec
each leg
p. 79

12
10 sec
each leg
p. 79

13
10 sec
each way
P. 82

14
10 sec
p. 81

Lift
25 mins

- Set = a fixed number of repetitions
- Rep = a repetition
- Use enough weight so last rep of set is slightly difficult
- Never lift to failure
- See Lifting Instructions, pp. 85–108

- Do these very carefully
- Do not do any stretch or exercise that causes pain
- Consult with your health professional

1
1 set
5–30 reps
each leg
p. 89

2
1 set
5–25 reps
each side
p. 89

3
1 set
5–25 reps
p. 91

4
1 set
5–25 reps
each leg
p. 91

5
1 set
5–25 reps
p. 90

6
1 set
5–25 reps
each leg
p. 90

7
1 set
5–25 reps
p. 86

8
1 set
5–25 reps
each leg
p. 87

Move

- Do anything that gets your heart rate up.
- See Moving Instructions, pp. 64–76

WALK
15 min

OR

SWIM
15 min

OR

TAI CHI
15 min

Photocopy this page and take it with you when you work out.

CANCER

The two most common causes of death for adults in this country are cardiovascular disease and various forms of cancer. By now, many people know that exercise is an important prescription in dealing with heart disease, but only recently have reports been coming in on the possibilities of preventing cancer by exercise and life-style changes. In fact, the medical community now estimates that most cancer cases are related to daily life-style habits.

Following are some basic facts about the most common types of cancer and recent discoveries of the beneficial effects of exercise and healthy diet.

THE TOP 15 PERSONAL CANCER-PREVENTION MEASURES

Two hundred leading cancer experts rated the following as the most valuable actions you can take in preventing cancer. They are listed in *order of importance*. (We don't agree with exercise being 13th on the list.)

1. Don't smoke or chew tobacco.
2. Get regular cancer screening tests.
3. Perform breast/testicular self-exams.
4. Limit sunlight exposure.
5. Avoid passive smoke.
6. Avoid high alcohol intake.
7. Reduce overall dietary fat.
8. Eat more food fiber.
9. Eat more fruits and vegetables.
10. Eat more whole-grain, high-fiber cereals.
11. Maintain normal weight.
12. Avoid household toxins.
13. Get regular exercise.
14. Limit exposure to nitrites.
15. Eat more cruciferous vegetables.

–*Body Bulletin* magazine

BAD NEWS, GOOD NEWS

The bad news is that the foods we eat, the amount of time we spend in the sun, cigarette and alcohol use, exposure to industrial chemicals, obesity, and many other factors contribute to risk of cancer. The good news is that exercise, good diet, and a healthy, active life-style can reduce the occurrence of certain cancers. For example, *The Physician and Sportsmedicine* magazine reported (in 1986) that out of the estimated 472,000 cancer deaths that year, 141,600 would be caused by tobacco use. Further, that numerous cancers of the colon, stomach, and esophagus are attributable to bad diet: high-fat and nitrite-cured foods and/or too much alcohol.

These causes of cancer can be controlled by the individual, so it only makes sense to cut down on the things that cause cancer and to implement changes, such as healthy diet and ongoing exercise, that will minimize cancer risk.

COLON CANCER

In a recent study, 8000 Japanese men living in Hawaii were examined and interviewed. Those who exercised had only ½ to ¾ the colon cancer risk compared to sedentary men in the study. This may have to do with the fact that exercise speeds up passage of food through the intestines, so carcinogens have a shorter exposure time and less chance to do damage. (Foods high in dietary fiber also reduce transit time through the intestines.) The relative risk of colon cancer also decreased as resting heart rate decreased.

Another study conducted by I-Min Lee of Harvard University had similar findings. In a study of some 17,000 male Harvard graduates conducted over 26 years, Lee reported that those who performed a minimum of two hours of aerobic exercise a week (or 10 miles of walking each week) had a 50% reduced incidence of colon cancer. Lee speculates that the same principles would apply to women.

OBESITY AND BREAST CANCER

Fitness may decrease the risk of breast cancer by reducing obesity, according to *Sports Medicine Digest* (January, 1991). Because fat cells make some estrogen, it is argued, reducing obesity cuts estrogen production and therefore the risk of breast cancer. Also, exercise appears to stimulate the immune system, which has a negative effect on the spread of cancer and helps prevent obesity.

FATS IN THE DIET

Too much fat in your diet will increase cancer risk. Dietary fat appears to encourage growth of cancer cells, primarily in the colon and breast. To cut down on dietary fat, avoid or minimize foods such as cream soups, desserts, ice cream, foods prepared with butter or margarine, cold cuts, and fast foods. It's also been shown that dark green vegetables and fruits contain certain dietary chemicals that help block cancer in the body.

FIBER IN THE DIET

The National Cancer Institute estimates that ⅓ of all cancer deaths may be related to diet. Studies conducted by the NCI suggest that eating foods high in fiber may reduce the risk of colon cancer. Americans now eat about 11 grams of fiber daily; the NCI recommends eating 20 to 30 grams daily, with a maximum of 35 grams. Fiber-rich foods such as whole grain breads, bran cereals, beans, fruits, and vegetables are preferable to fiber supplements. (*See fiber content of various foods, p. 132.*)

It is now known that about 80% of all cancers are related to environmental and life-style causes and that many of these cancers can be prevented through adoption of healthy practices.

–Diet and Cancer
Statement from National Cancer Institute, Bethesda, MD

. . . regular physical activity can reduce a woman's risk of developing premeno-pausal breast cancer by as much as 60%.

–Jane E Brody
The New York Times

Physically fit men die four times less often from cancer, and physically fit women die 16 times less often from cancer than unfit men and women.

–Dr. Steven Blair, Dr. Harold W. Kohl, et al.
"Physical Fitness and All-Cause Mortality," *Journal of the American Medical Association,* November, 1989

SMOKING

Cigarette smoking causes 30 percent of all cancer deaths in the United States. What if you're a smoker who wants to begin exercising? First of all, when you start an exercise program, expect immediate improvement in your cardiorespiratory health. Additionally, exercising will discourage you from smoking. How? When you start increasing your heart rate, your body will feel the damage smoke does to lungs and circulation. Exercising also helps reduce the stress that invariably goes along with quitting smoking.

While smoking has been a highly publicized risk for some 30 years, it is only within the last 10 years that so-called passive smoking (exposure to other people's smoke in enclosed spaces) has been recognized as a significant factor in risk of cancer.

(See section on smoking, pp. 181–182.)

ALCOHOL

Excessive alcohol intake can lead to many health problems. Whereas alcohol in moderation seems negligible in risk, heavy drinking is linked to cancers of the liver, throat, and mouth. Smokers who drink are giving themselves a double-dosed risk of cancer. Alcoholic drinks are also low in vitamins and minerals, high in calories, and very dehydrating.

EXERCISE AND CANCER

Exercise is a potent anti-cancer strategy. It reduces stress, helps control weight, and contributes to a more positive outlook. A good exercise program will lead to an improved overall life-style, which is one of the best ways of minimizing risk of cancer.

SUN EXPOSURE AND SKIN CANCER

To prevent cancer, it appears that avoiding excessive sun exposure is just as important as avoiding both alcohol and tobacco. "Nearly all of the more than 500,000 cases of non-melanoma skin cancer each year are caused by too much sun," said Paul E. Engstrom, M.D., of the Fox-Chase Cancer Center in Philadelphia. "The good news is that non-melanomas are highly treatable, so considerably fewer cancer deaths are attributable to sun exposure." The bad news is that excessive sun exposure seems to cause melanomas, which are rarer, but deadlier. The bottom line: Stay out of the sun when possible and when you can't, wear a protective hat and clothing and use sun-block.

RECOMMENDED READING

Call the *Cancer Information Service,* 800–4–CANCER for information

Choices in Healing: Integrating the Best of Conventional and Complimentary Approaches to Cancer by Michael Lerner ©1994. The MIT Press, Cambridge, MA.

Commonweal offers resources, referral information, and week-long residential programs for people with cancer interested in exploring complimentary therapies and pathways to healing. P. O. Box 316, Bolinas, CA 94924, 415-868-9017.

CARPAL TUNNEL SYNDROME

Between 1988 and 1992, the number of cumulative stress injuries in the United States soared 144% to 282,000.

San Francisco Chronicle

Recently, there's been growing awareness of a type of injury that affects office workers, especially those who use computers. Although these injuries are not on the same scale as some medical problems (like high blood pressure, arthritis, or cancer), they are unfortunately a persistent fact of life for many workers.

They are called *repetitive motion,* or *cumulative stress injuries* and tend to afflict people who do repetitive things with their hands. Although they affect both blue collar and white collar workers alike, the recent proliferation of computers in offices has called national attention to the problem. The Bureau of Labor Statistics reports that 63% of all workplace illnesses in 1992 were cumulative stress injuries. In fact, according to *Technology Review,* carpal tunnel syndrome repair is now the second-most-frequent surgical procedure performed in the United States.

THE NATURE OF THE PROBLEM

Unlike sudden injuries like broken bones or a lower back injury caused by lifting something too heavy, cumulative stress injuries result from a gradual, continual accumulation of small, sometimes unnoticeable changes that eventually produce pain. Often this type of process impinges on nerves or damages tissues as a result of a person's performing repetitious tasks, or from awkward positioning of the hand, leg, arm, or back for an extended period of time. Working at a computer keyboard seems to be responsible for the growing number of complaints, injuries, and lost work days in the office.

CARPAL TUNNEL SYNDROME

Carpal tunnel syndrome is named after the carpal bones in the wrist.

The carpal tunnel is a narrow space formed by bones and a ligament at the base of the palm, just above the wrist. Through that tunnel passes:

- The median nerve, which transmits sensation to the thumb and most of the fingers
- The tendons that operate the muscles of the hand

Tendons

Carpal ligament (forms roof of carpal tunnel)

Median nerve

TYPEWRITERS VS. COMPUTERS

In the days before word processors, typists did a greater variety of manual tasks — making corrections by hand, rolling a sheet of paper in and out of the carriage, manually returning the carriage, changing ribbons. This allowed the hands to move in a variety of

For some people, carpal tunnel syndrome is no more than a minor annoyance. Others experiencing it cannot sleep at night or open a jar.

directions and the brief pauses gave the wrists a rest. With computers, however, all this activity is automated. The operator may perform over 20,000 keystrokes in a single work period, with no variation and no "wrist rest" time.

WHEN THE NERVE IS DAMAGED

Continued bending of the wrist, especially in an unnatural position, can cause the tendons to swell and press on the very sensitive median nerve that runs through the carpal tunnel. Someone said it is like "stepping on a hose with water coming out."

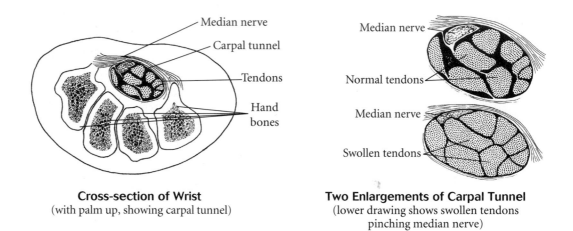

Cross-section of Wrist
(with palm up, showing carpal tunnel)

Two Enlargements of Carpal Tunnel
(lower drawing shows swollen tendons pinching median nerve)

In time, pressure atrophies the nerve and the muscles of the thumb and first three fingers that the nerve controls. This can result in numbness, loss of dexterity, and "pins and needles" in the hand that keep you awake at night. If the damage goes unchecked for too long, it can be permanent and, in fact, carpal tunnel damage has forced many people to change jobs.

AN OUNCE OF PREVENTION

If you have the type of job likely to cause these problems, but don't have this injury now, you can try to prevent this problem before it occurs by doing the exercises listed below or those shown on p. 158.

REMEDIES FOR CARPAL TUNNEL SYNDROME

- Vary the position of your wrists at work. Try not to work with them in a bent position.
- Take frequent breaks from the keyboard.
- Investigate *ergonomics,* or the study of how people adapt to the workplace. A new design in tables or chairs may alleviate the problem. (*See p. 163.*)
- An anti-inflammatory drug like aspirin may help.
- Wrap wrist(s) in ice packs to reduce swelling.

- Raise arms overhead and move arms in circles for a few minutes. Or dangle hands at sides and shake, with wrists loose. The aim is to restore circulation.

- Squeeze fingers, then stretch them out several times. Or squeeze a tennis ball.

- Special braces with built-in aluminum splints and Velcro fasteners that stop the wrist from bending can be worn at night and on the job whenever possible. They are available in most drug stores.

- You may need to take a week or two of rest, perhaps with your wrist in a splint.

- Surgery is a last resort. There are two types. "Open-hand" surgery is where an incision is made in both palm and wrist. This operation requires a lengthy recuperative period. In the newer technique, "closed-hand" surgery, only a local anesthetic is used to make a ¾-inch incision through which the surgeon will divide the carpal ligament with a special tool. A 2- to 6-week recovery period is typical for this procedure. Neither type of surgery, however, cures all cases, especially if the damage has gone unchecked for too long.

See the next page for wrist exercises.

OTHER REPETITIVE MOTION INJURIES

Other medical problems, such as thumb or wrist tendinitis, arthritis of the thumb, or thoracic outlet syndrome affect various body parts and can be caused by or aggravated by cumulative stress injuries. In many cases, paying attention to how you stand or sit as you work and varying or altering the position of your hands, wrists, arms, legs, and neck can alleviate the problem. Take stretching breaks every so often. Walk on a coffee break. If pain persists, see your family physician, occupational therapist (who will be quite familiar with these disorders, or a physiatrist (a nonsurgical doctor specializing in rehabilitation).

RECOMMENDED READING

Repetitive Strain Injury — A Computer User's Guide by Emil Pascarelli, M.D., and Deborah Quilter © 1993. Wiley Publishers, New York, NY.

Conquering Carpal Tunnel Syndrome by Sharon J. Butler © 1995. Advanced Press, Berwyn, PA. 800-909-9795.

Computer and Desk Stretches. Laminated 8½ x 11-inch card that fits in desk drawer. Program of stretches to do at your desk. Stretching, Inc., Palmer Lake, CO.

Computer Stretches. IBM-compatible software stretching program that "pops up" on computer screen at timed intervals. Stretching, Inc., Palmer Lake, CO.

AliMed Ergonomic Products—Large catalog of wrist straps, many other ergonomic office products. Dedham, MA. 800-225-2610.

Upper Extremity Technology Products Catalog contains a number of books on repetitive motion injuries, ergonomic design, rehabilitation, etc. "By therapists . . . for therapists." UE Tech, 2001 Blake Ave., 2-A, Glenwood Springs, CO 81601. 800-736-1894.

WRIST EXERCISES FOR CARPAL TUNNEL SYNDROME

WRIST EXTENSION AND FLEXION
EASY

Lay your arm on its side across a tabletop with your hand in a fist. Slowly bend your wrist forward and back. To measure your progress, trace on a piece of paper how far your hand extends in each direction when you bend your wrist.

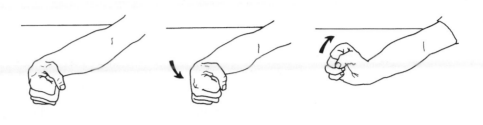

WRIST EXTENSION AND FLEXION
MODERATE

Lay your arm (palm down) on a tabletop with your wrist just over the edge. Slowly let your wrist bend down; then bend it back straight. Next, turn your forearm so that your palm is facing up and repeat the exercises.

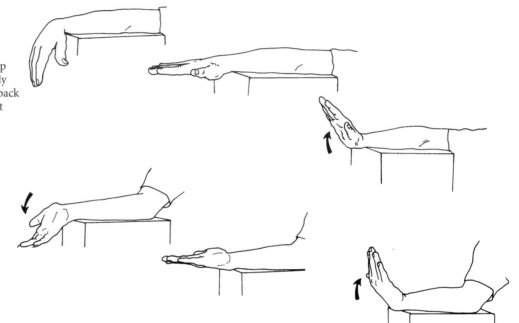

WRIST ADDUCTION AND ABDUCTION
EASY

Lay your arm flat across a tabletop, palm down. Slowly alternate stretching your thumb side of your hand to your forearm, then your little finger side of your hand to your forearm. To measure your progress, trace on a piece of paper how far your hand extends in each direction when you bend your wrist.

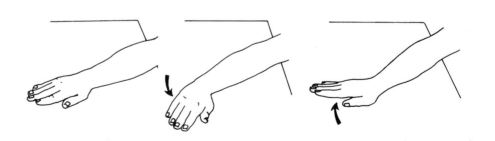

HAND ADDUCTION AND ABDUCTION
MODERATE

Lay your arm (palm down) on a tabletop with your wrist just over the edge. Slowly alternate stretching your thumb to your forearm, then your little finger to your forearm. Then turn your forearm so that your palm is facing up and repeat the exercises.

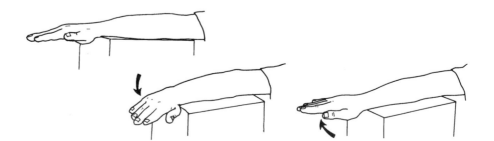

DIABETES

Diabetes mellitus is a chronic disorder of the metabolism of sugar, protein, and fat. Approximately 5 million Americans have known diabetes, and it is estimated that an equal number are undiagnosed.

TWO TYPES OF DIABETES

There are two types of diabetes:

- *Type I:* Formerly called *juvenile diabetes,* Type I represents 5 to 10% of all cases of diabetes and primarily affects people below the age of 30 (although it can be found at any age). This type requires insulin injections.
- *Type II:* Formerly called *adult-onset* diabetes. About 80% of those afflicted with diabetes have this type. It is strongly associated with obesity. Insulin injections are not required.

THE MISSING LINK

Although most diabetics know that insulin and diet are important in controlling diabetes, many are not aware of the importance of a third element: *exercise.* It's admittedly easier to take extra medication or to eat a good meal than it is to add exercise to your overall program. Many medical experts feel that diabetes treatment is less effective without exercise.

HOW THE BODY IS POWERED

To help you understand how physical activity helps control diabetes, let's look at the process by which our bodies convert fuel to energy for exercise, and what happens when insulin is missing.

Energy comes mainly from carbohydrates and fats stored in the body's cells. (Protein is not a preferred fuel for exercise.) These cells act as reservoirs in your body — they are depleted after you exercise and refilled after you eat.

When you begin to exercise, your body is fueled at first by carbohydrates. Carbohydrates are available from the bloodstream and can be released from stores in the liver when needed and transported to the muscles for energy.

THE ROLE OF INSULIN

Glucose (carbohydrates) cannot diffuse into the muscle without the help of insulin. Insulin is produced in the pancreas and binds with the insulin receptors on the muscle membrane. This allows glucose to pass through the cell membrane easily. However, insulin is absent in Type I diabetes and less effective in Type II diabetes. With little or no insulin available, glucose begins to increase in the bloodstream, with excess amounts spilling over into the urine.

Physically fit women have diabetes 66% less than unfit women.

–Dr. Rose Frisch
Harvard School of Public Health

THE ROLE OF EXERCISE

Exercise has an insulin-like effect on the muscles, it increases the permeability of the muscle membrane and the body's sensitivity to insulin. As a result, it reduces the amount of insulin needed for transport. The effect of exercise is to lower the amount of glucose in the blood, which is the main objective in controlling diabetes.

RISKS OF EXERCISE FOR TYPE I DIABETICS

Type I diabetics usually find that the more they exercise, the less insulin (injections) they require. Recent studies in humans (as well as animals) indicate that exercising the muscles into which insulin has been injected speeds its absorption into the bloodstream. However, Type I diabetics should consult their physicians about the proper ways to exercise and be aware of the following risks:

- Anyone who has high blood pressure or eye complications as a result of diabetes must be extra careful.

- Exercise is not recommended for Type I diabetics unless they are "under control". Diabetic control means being able to predictably regulate blood sugar. If blood sugar is too high, and exercise makes it go higher, there is risk of diabetic coma. If blood sugar is too low, the person risks hypoglycemia and may go into insulin shock. Diabetic control means balancing insulin, food intake, and exercise.

- Many doctors recommend that the Type I diabetic not inject insulin into the *active* muscles (the legs of a jogger, for example), if exercise is planned immediately after the injection; the accelerated absorption of the insulin into the bloodstream caused by exercise may make blood sugar more difficult to predict.

- Type I diabetics should exercise with a partner and always carry a source of carbohydrates.

EXERCISE, BODY FAT, AND TYPE II DIABETICS

For Type II diabetics, exercise is highly desirable, and lacks many of the dangers faced by Type I people. Since most Type IIs are overweight, exercise should focus on caloric expenditure. By losing weight, Type IIs can increase the number of insulin receptors on their body cells and thus improve the internal action of their own insulin. This will in turn help blood sugar return to normal, so less or no oral medication is necessary.

THE ROLE OF FOOD

If you have diabetes, you should go into each exercise session with a slightly elevated blood glucose level. You can do so by eating a carbohydrate snack about 30 minutes before beginning exercise.

The key to controlling diabetes is to maintain a consistent balance among:
- Insulin
- Exercise
- Diet

BODY FAT AND TYPE I DIABETICS

Increased levels of body fat reduce the body's sensitivity to insulin; thus, more insulin is needed to help blood glucose enter the muscles. Exercise can help those with excess body fat and diabetes reach an ideal weight. By lowering your body weight, you reduce your dependence on injections and you generally feel fitter and healthier.

EXERCISE PROGRAMS FOR DIABETICS

See The Program Before the Program, pp. 15–18.

RECOMMENDED READING

Diabetes and Exercise: Guidelines for Safe and Enjoyable Activity by Marion Franz © 1988. International Diabetes Center, 5000 W. 39th St., Minneapolis MN 55416

The Diabetic's Guide to Health and Fitness by Kris Berg © 1986. Human Kinetics, Champaign, IL.

The Energetic Diabetic by Neil Armstrong and Diane Wahot © 1985. Brady Communications Corporation, Bowie, MD.

THE DIGITAL WORKPLACE

ELECTRONIC STRESS

An estimated 50 million Americans work on computers. While the advantages to employers are undisputed, the disadvantages and even dangers for employees are just now being recognized:

- To increase efficiency and to gather a greater amount of data on each transaction, many offices have broken jobs down into simpler, less challenging tasks that require less decision-making. Elements of factory assembly-line work have crept into clerical jobs. More rote decisions, less creative input.

- Human interaction with co-workers and supervisors has been replaced by interaction with, and evaluation by, machines. There is less give and take, less personal human contact, less social interaction.

- With an electronic keyboard, monitor, and printer, much less movement is required. Instead of manually inserting and removing stationery and envelopes into a typewriter, keyboarded data is automatically relayed to the printer. Also, so many tasks can be keyboarded, and such close attention to the monitor is required, that the operator tends to sit very still and move around very little.

- Along with segmented, assembly-line type clerical work and lack of personal contact comes emotional stress. "The same things that cause repetitive-motion injuries cause (emotional) stress injuries," says Charley Richardson, director of the University of Lowell's technology and work program in Massachusetts. "People get put in boxes, can't move around, can't use their skills. It's not good for them."

CARPAL TUNNEL SYNDROME

Carpal tunnel syndrome and other repetitive motion injuries have increased greatly in the last decade. (290,000 cases of repetitive motion injuries were reported in 1989, a sevenfold increase since 1981.) A recent survey by California's occupational health program suggested that the actual frequency of carpal tunnel syndrome — a type of repetitive motion injury common among computer operators — is some 50 times greater than the number reported to state officials. (*See pp. 155–157 for a more complete discussion of this problem.*)

TELECOMMUTING

Telecommuting refers to working at home rather than the office. It's been made possible by personal computers, modems, and other electronic technology. Employees can maintain contact with employers via phone and modem.

- *Advantages:* reduced commute time and cost, casual dress, flexibility of work hours, greater ability to concentrate, and increased productivity.

- *Disadvantages:* isolation from co-workers, distractions in the home environment, reduction of living space, and the possibility of burning out.

Experience over the past several years seems to indicate that telecommuting works best on a part-time basis: that is, the employee goes into the office one or more days a week. Contact is maintained with co-workers and supervisors and the telecommuter does not become too isolated.

Some problems of telecommuting, such as operating an electronic keyboard, are the same at home as in the office: lack of movement and/or use of the muscles, which leads to stiffness, loss of muscular strength, and other ailments attributable to the sedentary life.

ERGONOMICS

Ergonomics is the science of providing office furniture, tools, and equipment that improve the comfort, safety, and health of the office worker. For example:

- *Desk.* Conventional desk surfaces are 29 inches high. A typical recommended height for computing surfaces is 26 inches from the floor.

- *Chair.* Your chair may be the most important piece of furniture in the office, so it pays to select one carefully. Special chairs with two control levers allow you not only to raise and lower the seat easily, but to tilt both the seat and backrest to any desired angle. They are in the $200 to $300 range, but well worth it for both employer (reduced health care costs) and employee.

- *Computer screen.* A rule of thumb is to sit at arm's length away from the screen.

- *Lighting.* Whether you use natural or electric light, direct it toward the side or behind your line of vision, not in front of or above your line of vision. Northern daylight is the best light for operating a computer, whether in the office or at home.

SAN FRANCISCO'S VDT LAW

In late 1990, San Francisco became the first major American city to pass a law aimed at protecting workers from the health and safety risks associated with video display terminals (VDTs). The legislation requires employers with 15 or more employees to provide safe VDT stations with state-of-the-art chairs, keyboards, lighting, and anti-glare screens. An advisory committee has been appointed to study and make recommendations on protecting VDT workers from possible radiation emissions.

EXERCISE AND ELECTRONICS

Electronic office technology is here to stay. In the future, more and more people will be operating computers and spending more time doing so. If you operate a computer, it's important for you to recognize (and research) all the problems associated with the digital workplace.

We recommend exercise as one of the most important factors in the life of any office worker, especially those who operate computers. Follow the general programs and philosophy in this book, take stretching breaks, and move around as much as possible during the work day. *(See the On the Job section on pp. 33–35 for stretches and exercises that can be done in the office.)* Doing so will minimize the health hazards of sitting for long periods at a keyboard in front of an electronic monitor.

RECOMMENDED READING

Sitting on the Job by Scott W. Donkin, D.C. © 1986. Houghton Mifflin, Boston, MA.

Computer and Desk Stretches. Laminated 8½ x 11-inch card that fits in desk drawer. Program of stretches to do at desk. Stretching, Inc., Palmer Lake, CO.

Stretching on the Job. Book with software stretching program that "pops up" on computer screen at timed intervals. Available in late 1995. Stretching, Inc., Palmer Lake, CO.

Telecommuting Review: The Gordon Report. (Meant for employers.) Gil Gordon Associates, 10 Donner Court, Monmouth Junction, NJ, 08852, 908-329-2266.

HIGH BLOOD PRESSURE

WHAT IS BLOOD PRESSURE?

Blood pressure is the force of blood against the walls of the arteries. This force is produced by your heart as it pumps blood through your arteries. With each heartbeat, the blood pressure in your arteries increases.

WHAT DO FIGURES LIKE 120/80 MEAN?

When your doctor gives you a blood pressure reading, it consists of two figures:

- *Systolic* blood pressure measures the pressure of blood in your arteries when your heart is beating. It's a measurement of how hard your heart works to pump blood. The first figure, 120 is considered normal.

- *Diastolic* blood pressure measures the pressure of blood on your arteries when your heart is at rest between beats. It's lower than the first number since it's measured when your heart is relaxed. The second figure, 80 is considered normal.

WHO IS MOST LIKELY TO DEVELOP HIGH BLOOD PRESSURE?

People with the following characteristics:

- Overweight
- Sedentary life-style
- High-stress life
- Family history of high blood pressure
- High salt intake

WHAT WILL EXERCISE DO FOR YOU?

Exercise can help control elevated blood pressure. Recently, it's been shown that physical activity may work as effectively as drugs in lowering high blood pressure. New studies show that regular exercise can reduce mild to moderate hypertension, without the symptoms that often accompany the use of medication.

EXERCISE VS. DRUGS

The *Journal of the American Medical Association* (May, 1990), reported a study of 52 men with mild hypertension (systolic pressure between 140–159 and diastolic between 90–104) . They were divided into three groups: the first group was given a drug called a *beta-blocker,* the second took a drug called a *calcium blocker,* and the third group took a *placebo*. All three groups then did a 10-week program of endurance and circuit weight training. Systolic blood pressure dropped as low in the placebo group as it did in the beta-blocker and calcium-blocker groups (an average of 14 points).

OPTIMUM BLOOD PRESSURE

A reading of 120/80 is optimum. Physicians generally conclude that the lower the pressure, the better.

HIGH BLOOD PRESSURE IN AMERICA

Approximately 58 million Americans have high blood pressure.

SALT SUBSTITUTES

Spice foods with natural low-sodium flavorings: lemon and lime juice, herbs and spices (like basil and oregano), and herb vinegars. Use chopped onion and garlic liberally.

Regular exercise helps reduce systemic arterial blood pressure.

–Dr. William Haskell
Heart Disease Prevention Program Stanford University Medical Center.

CUT BACK ON SALT

Researchers have recently found that salt has a greater link to high blood pressure than was previously thought. As reported in the *British Medical Journal*, a review of 78 studies involving some 47,000 people clearly indicated the benefits of a low-salt diet. A comparison of salt-eating industrialized societies with primitive societies that do not use much salt showed that those who used more salt had higher blood pressure. Dr. Malcolm Law, who directed the study, said that, "Everyone, even if their doctor didn't tell them they were at high risk for heart disease, should reduce the salt in their diets by at least three grams (half a teaspoon) a day."

EXERCISE VS. NO EXERCISE

Moderate exercise in itself reduces blood pressure. Researchers at the University of Arizona had 14 men and women with mild hypertension participate in a 12-month walking program, walking 3 days a week at 50 percent maximum heart rate. Another group of 12 served as controls by not exercising. The walkers lowered their blood pressure by an average of 9 points.

A 5-year study at Northwestern Medical School of 200 hypertension-prone Chicago workers was reported in *The Physician and Sportsmedicine*. Hypertension occurred in 8.8 percent of the group that exercised and in 19.2 percent of the group that did not.

WHAT TO DO?

If you're one of the 58 million Americans with high blood pressure, consult your doctor about starting an exercise program. If you are not, why wait until you have developed mild or high blood pressure before starting an exercise program? Walking, stair climbing, swimming, and cycling are excellent activities for reducing blood pressure.

WEIGHT TRAINING AND HIGH BLOOD PRESSURE

Because weight training can cause blood pressure to increase greatly, physicians for years were reluctant to prescribe it for patients with high blood pressure. Recently, thanks to a number of studies, however, resistance training has been shown to reduce diastolic blood pressure, as well as to increase HDL cholesterol (the "good" type) and increase insulin sensitivity. As reported in *The Physician and Sportsmedicine* (June 1991): "Newer evidence is proving the safety and benefit of weight training, specifically of programs with moderate resistance and relatively high repetition."

EXERCISE REDUCES STRESS

People who work out find that regular exercise helps increase their resistance to stress. They tend not to overreact to daily hassles and are more relaxed after exercising. Improved stress response will lead to better blood pressure response as well. Learning to relax for short periods of time during the workday is extremely helpful.

Exercise, along with weight loss and reduction in salt intake and alcohol, will also help fight other lifestyle disorders, such as diabetes, heart disease, and obesity. Moderate exercise and regular activity can be important assets in reaching your blood pressure goal and staying fit.

EXERCISE PROGRAMS

For a gentle exercise program, see pp. 15–18, but be sure to consult with your doctor before starting any type of exercise program. Be careful of any type of exercise where blood flow is restricted, such as holding your breath while weight training. Also, be careful of strenuous chores, such as shoveling snow.

RECOMMENDED READING

Overcoming Hypertension by Kenneth H. Cooper © 1990. Bantam, New York, NY.

HIGH CHOLESTEROL AND HEART DISEASE

WHAT IS CHOLESTEROL?

Cholesterol is a waxy, fatty substance that is both produced in your body and introduced in your diet through animal-based foods. Despite its killer reputation, some cholesterol is needed for certain vital body functions — it is transported in the blood and it helps in building cell walls and making hormones.

SO WHAT'S THE PROBLEM?

The problem is *excess* cholesterol. When there's too much in your system, it continues to circulate in the bloodstream and may sooner or later be deposited on the inner walls of your arteries. There, it can thicken and harden, narrowing the passages through which the blood must flow.

When this happens, it's like sludge deposits in an old pipe, and it's called *atherosclerosis,* or "hardening of the arteries." There can be two serious results of this condition:

1. A *heart attack,* when a blood clot gets stuck in an artery leading to the heart
2. A *stroke,* when a clot lodges in an artery leading to the brain

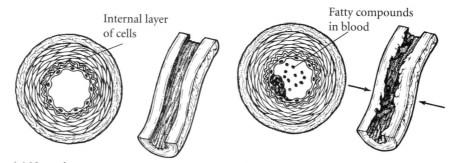

(a) Normal

(b) Fatty compound may be deposited in susceptible cells, forming a plaque

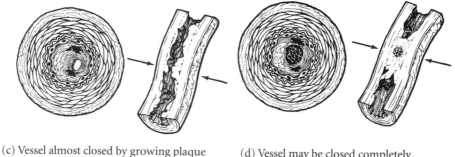

(c) Vessel almost closed by growing plaque in which calcium has been deposited

(d) Vessel may be closed completely. Hemorrhage may occur

Normal Artery and Three Stages of Progressive Closure from Excess Fat in Diet

HEART DISEASE IS A KILLER

Coronary heart disease is the number one cause of death in America today, outnumbering deaths from cancer and accidents combined. More than 500,000 people die of heart attacks every year and over 5 million Americans have angina or other heart problems.

HOW DO YOU MEASURE CHOLESTEROL?

Cholesterol is measured by a blood test. If you are over 20 years old, here are some commonly accepted risk factors:

- Desirable: under 200 mg/dl (milligrams per deciliter)
- Borderline-high risk: 200–239 mg/dl
- High risk: 240 mg/dl or above

BLOOD WILL TELL

Moreover, there's more to the tests than just the "mg/dl" total cholesterol figures:

- *LDLs* (low-density lipoproteins) = "the bad guys." These carry cholesterol to the body cells. The higher the level of LDLs, the worse it is.
- *HDLs* (high density lipoproteins) = "the good guys." These remove cholesterol from the blood by bringing it back to the liver where it is broken down and excreted.
- *Triglycerides* = fatty molecules in the blood. High levels are not good.

Interpreting a blood test is too complex to cover here. We recommend *Controlling Cholesterol* by Dr. Kenneth Cooper *(see p. 171)* for recommended levels and for other pertinent information about blood tests.

Regular exercise reduces harmful LDL cholesterol while increasing beneficial HDL cholesterol.

–Dr. Joseph Patsch
Newsweek, August 1984

THE IMPORTANCE OF EXERCISE

Regular exercise affects the risk factors relating to heart attacks and strokes in several ways:

- It burns calories and helps cut down body fat deposits.
- It lowers total cholesterol level.
- It increases the HDL ("good") cholesterol level.
- It helps to decrease the clumping of platelets in the bloodstream that starts clots. Exercise significantly increases the output of an enzyme that helps prevent platelets from "sticking" together.

EXERCISE VS. ASPIRIN

As we've pointed out, blood clots forming inside blood vessels can lead to heart attacks and strokes. Until recently, one of the few things doctors could recommend was taking an aspirin every day or every other day. Recent studies, however, show that not only will vigorous exercise help the body dissolve blood clots naturally, but can also help prevent new clots from forming.

THE IMPORTANCE OF DIET

You most likely know that the American diet contains way too much fat. Daily cholesterol intake should be reduced from the current average of about 450 mg to no more than 100 to 300 milligrams. Dietary cholesterol is found only in animal fat, such foods as whole milk, eggs, cheese, fatty meats, and ice cream. Dietary saturated fat, even though it may contain no cholesterol, should also be reduced because it serves as the primary raw material used by the liver to produce cholesterol in the body.

The typical American diet is about 40% fat, most of it coming from saturated fat. The American Heart Association recommends that we reduce our total fat intake to less than 30%; saturated fat should make up only about one-third of total fat intake. Lastly, increasing your fiber intake and maintaining a sensible body weight will help control cholesterol levels. *(See the chapter on food, pp. 127–136 for more information on this topic.)*

READING LABELS IS TRICKY

In 1991, the Food and Drug Administration began cracking down on food companies claiming on labels that their product contained low or no cholesterol. Then-FDA commissioner David A. Kesseler said he was particularly concerned about labels that display heart symbols and imply that they prevent heart disease. No-cholesterol products might have other fats that could lead to high cholesterol and heart illness, he pointed out.

CAN THIN PEOPLE EAT MORE FAT?

Many fit-minded people think they can eat whatever they want so long as they exercise regularly. Pass the butter! Bring on the ice cream! This is a mistaken and sometimes deadly notion. No one, fat or thin, should load up on fats. A person can appear healthy and lean on the outside, but have internal clogging of the arteries from a high-fat diet. (Heredity also plays a role.)

Endurance athletes who eat high saturated fat diets often have dangerously high LDL (the bad) cholesterol levels.

> *Cholesterol is not a fuel that the body can burn off.*

WEIGHT LOSS (TEMPORARILY) INCREASES CHOLESTEROL

People who lose a lot of weight may see a temporary rise in cholesterol. This probably occurs when fat stores release cholesterol into the blood as pounds are shed. In a study at the University of California at Davis, 6 obese women who lost an average of 67 pounds in 5 to 7 months on a very low-calorie diet first experienced a drop in blood cholesterol. About 6 months after the women began their diets, blood cholesterol rose. It finally dropped again after the women maintained their weight loss for 2 months or more.

EXERCISE FOR PEOPLE WITH HIGH CHOLESTEROL

Show your physician the programs on pp. 16–18 to see if they would be acceptable as a basis for you to start exercising.

RECOMMENDED READING

Controlling Cholesterol by Kenneth Cooper, M.D. © 1988. Bantam Books, New York, NY.

The New Fit or Fat by Covert Bailey © 1991. Houghton Mifflin, New York, NY.

The Pritikin Promise by Nathan Pritikin © 1991. Pocket Books, New York, NY.

Dr. Dean Ornish's Program for Reversing Heart Disease by Dr. Dean Ornish © 1990. Random House, New York, NY.

OSTEOPOROSIS

Osteoporosis is a painful disease characterized by weak, brittle, porous bones that tend to fracture easily. According to the National Osteoporosis Foundation, more than 24 million Americans currently suffer from this condition. Most are elderly women whose bone mass has dropped significantly after menopause.

OSTEOPOROSIS IN WOMEN AND MEN

Osteoporosis strikes 8 times as many women as it does men. Nearly half of all American women over 65 suffer from osteoporosis to some extent, and one-third of women over 65 suffer vertebral fractures. The main reason seems to be that after menopause, loss of estrogen accelerates calcium loss in the body.

One of the most familiar signs of osteoporosis is the rounded back posture known as "dowager's hump," which comes about when the spinal column weakens and individual vertebrae collapse due to "crush fractures." The spine then develops a noticeable curve, and this condition causes pain and loss of height.

If a woman has had her ovaries removed, the chances of getting osteoporosis are significantly increased. Also, if your mother or grandmother became stooped or suffered fractures of the hips and wrists, your chances of developing osteoporosis are greater.

Presently, the United States population aged 65 or older is about 12%. But that percentage is expected to double in the next 30 years, which means a growing problem in this country for men as well as women.

SOME FACTS ON BONES

People tend to think of bones as rigid, inanimate structures. Not true! Bones are made of living, growing tissue. At the center of some bones is the soft red marrow where red blood cells and many of the immune system cells originate. The external covering of the bones consists of a hard outer shell, where calcium — the most abundant mineral in the body — is stored.

Some 99 percent of the body's calcium is stored in the bones and teeth. For one thing, it gives bones their unique strength. But calcium has other important functions. It regulates the pumping of the heart, sends nerve signals to the brain, helps muscles contract, and assists in various other essential operations.

If there is not enough calcium in the bloodstream to carry out all of the tasks just mentioned and others, the body will borrow from the bones. Thus, too little calcium in the diet can weaken bones.

PREVENTING OSTEOPOROSIS

The best way for women to prevent osteoporosis is to build strong bones before their 30s, so that they will have heavy bone mass through the menopausal years and beyond. But no matter what your age, preventive measures can be helpful:

- Make sure your diet contains 1200 milligrams of calcium per day, either through food, or supplements, or both. Calcium is needed for strong bone growth.

- Estrogen replacement may be recommended by your physician if you have had your ovaries removed or had early menopause. Estrogen is used by the body to help transport calcium into your bones. However, we'd advise you to make a careful study of the effects of estrogen — in the 1970s it was discovered that estrogen users had a much higher risk of cancer of the lining of the uterus. In more recent years, doctors lowered the dosages of estrogen and combined it with another female hormone, progesterone, to minimize this risk. A study published in the *New England Journal of Medicine* showed a higher risk of breast cancer for women taking these two drugs.

- Both smoking and high alcohol intake increase the risk of osteoporosis. Smokers tend to have lower estrogen levels and excess alcohol is often accompanied by poor nutrition, so moderating, or ceasing either of these activities will improve matters.

- Frequent radical dieting tends to increase the risk of osteoporosis. If there is calcium missing in the diet, the bones will release calcium for other critical bodily functions.

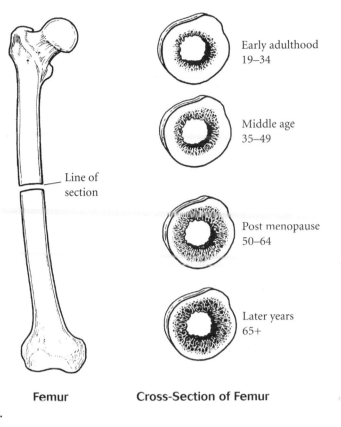

Line of section

Femur

Cross-Section of Femur

Early adulthood 19–34

Middle age 35–49

Post menopause 50–64

Later years 65+

THE ROLE OF EXERCISE IN PREVENTING OSTEOPOROSIS

We previously pointed out that bones are composed of living tissue. And just like muscles, tendons, and ligaments, bones respond to demands placed on them. When bones are stressed by physical activity, they respond by getting stronger.

The effects of exercise on bone strength became an issue when the first astronauts came back from space. Physicians at NASA found evidence of measurable bone loss even after just a short time in space. This finding led some scientists to speculate that the "use it or lose it" principle was in effect, that when the bones were not stressed, they began to weaken.

WHAT TYPE OF EXERCISE?

A modest program is recommended for older women who want stronger bones, as well as for younger women who are working towards reaching a high "peak bone mass" in their mid-30s. The key is that exercise must be *weight-bearing* in nature.

Weight-bearing exercises include activities such as walking, jogging, jumping rope, dancing, racquet sports, cross-country skiing, and low-impact aerobics. Swimming, cycling, and yoga are healthy activities, but are not generally thought of as weight-bearing.

STAY ACTIVE

Many doctors encourage patients with osteoporosis to remain as physically active as possible, but to avoid activities where one might fall and break a bone.

Walking is highly recommended. If you are able to be up and around, do so — the worst thing you can do is to give in and take to your bed or chair. Lack of physical activity is harmful, not only physically, but psychologically as well.

CALCIUM *CAN* STOP BONE LOSS IN OLDER WOMEN

General agreement has always held that it's wise for premenopausal women to ensure they are getting enough calcium so that enough gets deposited in the bones prior to age-related bone loss. Young women are advised to make sure they are getting 1200 milligrams of calcium daily as insurance against excess bone loss, and some health professionals today recommend 1500 milligrams for post-menopausal women.

Likewise, there seemed to be — until recently — widespread agreement that extra calcium in the diet couldn't prevent bone loss in older, post-menopausal women. But in a Tufts University study, published in late 1990 in the *New England Journal of Medicine*, it was determined that calcium supplements *did* help prevent bone loss in post-menopausal women, especially those who previously had been taking in less than the RDA of 800 milligrams daily.

HOW TO GET ENOUGH CALCIUM

Calcium is a mineral required by our bodies for life. Calcium must come from the diet; our bodies cannot make it. Calcium-rich foods include dairy products, soy products, sesame seeds, and green vegetables like broccoli, green leafy vegetables, and especially collard greens. Many people are interested in calcium supplements to insure adequate daily intake, but some of the supplements have had problems — some have not been soluble enough to be broken down and dispersed in the bloodstream. Some, like those containing bone meal or dolomite, sometimes have high levels of lead or other toxins. A relatively new patented supplement, calcium citrate malate, added to fruit juices, seems to overcome many of the problems associated with other calcium supplements. A combination of dairy products and calcium carbonate supplements in pill form seems to work well. Note that calcium taken *with* food is more readily absorbed by the body.

EXERCISE PROGRAM FOR PEOPLE WITH OSTEOPOROSIS

The right type and amount of exercise depend upon your age and condition. Consult your physician and refer to pp. 15–18. Or, if you are already exercising, see the Circuit Training programs on pp. 45–47.

RECOMMENDED READING:

The Tufts University Guide to Total Nutrition © 1991. Harper Collins, New York, NY.

Jane Brody's Nutrition Book — A Lifetime Guide to Good Eating and Better Health and Weight Control by Jane Brody © 1981. W.W. Norton, New York, NY.

The McDougall Plan by John A. McDougall, M.D., and Mary A. McDougall © 1983. New Win Publishing, Clinton, NJ.

OVERWEIGHT

See Program for Weight Management, p. 178.

The number of overweight American adults has risen to nearly two out of three, and almost a third of those who are too heavy don't admit it.

–Associated Press

We've titled this section *overweight*, but what we're really concerned with is *obesity*. Too often the terms are used interchangeably.

Overweight refers to body weight in excess of known standards. Today, the standards most often used are the Metropolitan Life Insurance Company height/weight charts.

Obesity, on the other hand, is defined in the medical dictionaries as an "... abnormal amount of fat on the body ... the term is not usually employed unless the person is 20 to 30% over average weight for his or her age, sex, and height."

We use the word *overweight* here because some people wouldn't read this if we titled it obesity. But it is obesity, or being *overfat,* that we're concerned with.

Weighing yourself on a scale only measures your weight, it doesn't tell you how fat you are. Standard height/weight charts can't tell you how much fat you're carrying. A football player might be considered overweight by the height/weight charts, but the weight is not fat, it's muscle.

At the other extreme, someone who sits most of the day may have too much fat and too little muscle, yet weigh within the standard chart guidelines.

RISKS OF OVERWEIGHT VS. OBESITY

Being a few pounds overweight generally poses no health risk, but obesity can contribute to high blood pressure, diabetes, arthritis, cancer, and heart disease. Obesity not only decreases life expectancy, but can cause psychological stress due to worry and lack of confidence in oneself.

COMMERCIAL DIETS

Unfortunately, most people who want to lose weight think in terms of dieting. It's quick, you just follow the directions, or consume the product, and the pounds melt off, right? This practice is reinforced by the number of fad diets, books, and TV ads that abound in America. (It's a billion dollar business!)

SCALE WORSHIP

A scale only gives you one number — your total body weight is meaningless unless you know how much is muscle and how much is fat.

QUICK WEIGHT LOSS

Most overweight people are looking for quick weight loss, but diets and dieters do not take into account that the excess pounds have accumulated slowly over the years (due to poor eating habits and lack of exercise); weight loss — permanent weight loss, that is — must likewise be a slow process.

THE IMPORTANCE OF FEELING GOOD

Shouldn't that be our goal? Not the perfect body — whatever that might be — but a body that feels and works well? The 250-pound body can be taught, just like any body, to move and become accomplished in a physical activity. The larger woman is not unhealthy just because she's heavy. She may be in much better shape — both physically and emotionally — than the thin woman who continually restricts food and uses exercise to control weight rather than having fun and living fully.

–Women's Sports & Fitness

WHY DIETS FAIL

The major reason many diets fail is, as mentioned, the urgency factor. We Americans want results. When we decide to make a change, we want it to happen now! And there always seem to be self-proclaimed experts waiting in the wings with the latest fad diet. It's funny how many M.D.s or Ph.D.s feel qualified to recommend the latest wonder diet that will let you lose 5 to 10 pounds a week, with only "moderate" changes in your lifestyle.

> *Quick Weight Loss = Quick Weight Gain*

How many of your friends have shed the pounds under the latest "miracle" program, only to eventually gain it all (and a little more) back? We won't belabor the point. Covert Bailey calls this up-and-down cycle of weight loss/gain ". . . the rhythm method of girth control."

METABOLISM AND DIET

Metabolism is the sum of energy your body requires. Metabolic *rate* is a measure of how fast you burn energy (calories). Strict dieting throws your metabolic rate into a tailspin. This process is thought to be a throwback to our ancient hunting and gathering ancestors: when the body is deprived of food, your metabolic rate slows way down. In prehistoric times, the body conserved its fat reserves for times of famine.

Fad dieting can also cause loss of muscle mass. When carbohydrate supplies are too low, the body literally feeds upon itself. Muscle protein is broken down as a source of fuel. On most quick diets, weight loss is mostly water and lost muscle; relatively little body fat is lost.

SO WHAT'S THE SOLUTION?

Exercise. Exercise helps keep metabolism at a steady level, even when you eat less. Exercise also helps maintain muscle mass when you diet. *Permanent weight control involves a lifelong commitment to regular exercise as well as good eating habits.* Whereas faddish diets and stop-and-start exercise programs ultimately end in disappointment, maintaining optimal body composition entails regular exercise and a diet based on sound nutritional knowledge. *(See discussion on Food, pp. 128–136.)*

EXERCISE IS A KEY INGREDIENT

With as little as 30 minutes of exercise, 3 days a week (equivalent to walking 5 to 6 miles a week), you can lose up to a quarter-pound of fat a week.

Doesn't sound like much? Well, in one year you could lose 12 to 15 pounds of fat from exercise alone. Eat a more healthy diet and the results will be even greater.

WEIGHT MANAGEMENT

Stretch every day.
Lift OR Move on alternate days.
This program will take 41 minutes.

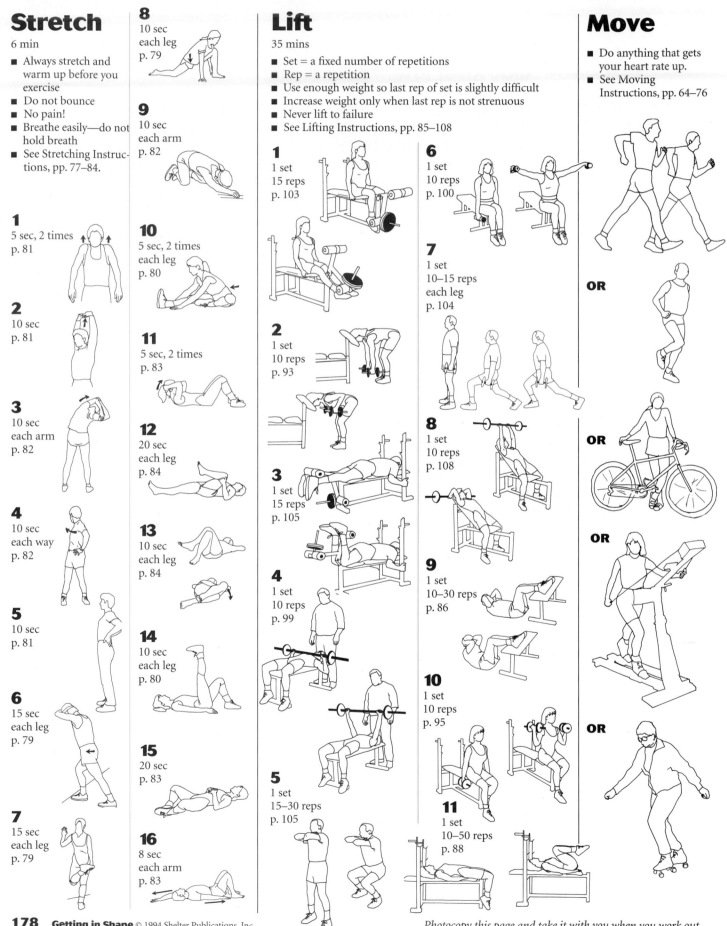

Stretch

6 min

- Always stretch and warm up before you exercise
- Do not bounce
- No pain!
- Breathe easily—do not hold breath
- See Stretching Instructions, pp. 77–84.

1 5 sec, 2 times p. 81

2 10 sec p. 81

3 10 sec each arm p. 82

4 10 sec each way p. 82

5 10 sec p. 81

6 15 sec each leg p. 79

7 15 sec each leg p. 79

8 10 sec each leg p. 79

9 10 sec each arm p. 82

10 5 sec, 2 times each leg p. 80

11 5 sec, 2 times p. 83

12 20 sec each leg p. 84

13 10 sec each leg p. 84

14 10 sec each leg p. 80

15 20 sec p. 83

16 8 sec each arm p. 83

Lift

35 mins

- Set = a fixed number of repetitions
- Rep = a repetition
- Use enough weight so last rep of set is slightly difficult
- Increase weight only when last rep is not strenuous
- Never lift to failure
- See Lifting Instructions, pp. 85–108

1 1 set 15 reps p. 103

2 1 set 10 reps p. 93

3 1 set 15 reps p. 105

4 1 set 10 reps p. 99

5 1 set 15–30 reps p. 105

6 1 set 10 reps p. 100

7 1 set 10–15 reps each leg p. 104

8 1 set 10 reps p. 108

9 1 set 10–30 reps p. 86

10 1 set 10 reps p. 95

11 1 set 10–50 reps p. 88

Move

- Do anything that gets your heart rate up.
- See Moving Instructions, pp. 64–76

OR

OR

OR

OR

Photocopy this page and take it with you when you work out.

WEIGHT TRAINING TO LOSE WEIGHT?

In 1991, *Fitness Management Magazine* conducted a study to determine the role of weight training on body composition changes. In this study, 72 overweight men and women were put into two groups. Both ate the same diets and exercised 30 minutes a day for 8 weeks. But one group followed a typical weight-loss exercise program, spending all 30 minutes on aerobic exercise, while the second group did 15 minutes of aerobic exercise (exercycling) and 15 minutes of weight training (Nautilus machines). Here are the results:

EXERCISE PROGRAM	N	BODY WEIGHT CHANGES	FAT WEIGHT CHANGES	MUSCLE WEIGHT CHANGES
Endurance exercise only	22	−3.5 pounds	−3.0 pounds	−0.5 pounds
Endurance and strength exercise	50	−8.0 pounds	−10.0 pounds	+2.0 pounds

WON'T EXERCISE INCREASE MY APPETITE?

High intensity exercise *will* stimulate your appetite. It lowers your blood glucose levels and your body will demand more food than normal.

But several recent studies have shown that *moderate* exercise tends to actually decrease appetite for several hours after your workout, the reason being that blood is directed away from the stomach to your working muscles. That's why taking a walk during your lunch break will help.

NO LOSS OF WEIGHT AT FIRST?

When you start an exercise program along with dietary changes to lose weight, it's important to understand the difference between fat loss and lean tissue loss. As you get older, if you do not exercise you lose lean tissue — mainly bone and muscle mass. This is especially true for people who sit most of the day.

But when you start to exercise you tend to gain lean weight (fat-free weight). Thus, when you start an exercise program, you may not lose weight on the scale for a few weeks, or even a few months. This is *normal,* and you shouldn't worry. Fat weight is being lost, but lean weight is being added at about the same rate. You're losing fat and gaining muscle, so don't sweat it!

Don't depend on the scale to chart your progress especially at first. Just look at yourself in the mirror. How do your clothes fit? Are good changes going on with your body shape or physique? Do you feel better?

ARE you FIT	or	FAT?
Fit people sink.		Fat people float.
Fit people are fat-burners.		Fat people are sugar-burners.
When fit people eat sugar, they make glycogen.		When fat people eat sugar, they make fat.
Fit people have lots of fat-burning enzymes.		Fat people have few fat-burning enzymes.
Fit people eat more than fat people.		Fat people diet and fast frequently, which lowers metabolic rate.
Fit people *use* fat efficiently.		Fat people *store* fat efficiently.
When fit people exercise, it is usually aerobic exercise.		When fat people exercise, it is often anaerobic exercise.
Fit people "waste" energy in everyday activities.		Fat people "conserve" energy throughout the day.
Fit people have long, lean, shapely muscles.		Fat people have short, round, fatty muscles.
Fit people can be overweight without being overfat.		Fat people can be overfat without being overweight.
Exercise decreases hunger in fit people.		Exercise triggers hunger in fat people.

Source: *The New Fit or Fat* by Covert Bailey, Houghton Mifflin, Boston, MA.

RECOMMENDED READING

Nutrition, Weight Control and Exercise by Frank I. Katch and William D. McArdle © 1988. Lea & Febiger, Philadelphia, PA.

The New Fit or Fat by Covert Bailey © 1991. Houghton Mifflin, Boston, MA.

Maximum Metabolism by Robert Giller, M.D., and Kathy Mathews © 1989. Berkeley Books, New York, NY.

The T-Factor Diet by Martin Katahn © 1990. Bantam, New York, NY.

SMOKING

In 1964, the Surgeon General's Report on Smoking and Health presented clear scientific evidence on the hazards of cigarette smoking. Today, over 30 years later, researchers have shown that smoking is even more dangerous than was first believed.

> *Smoking is the number one preventable cause of death in America.*

The more you smoke, the greater your danger of heart attack or death. (Other risk factors being equal, the average smoker is twice as likely to have a heart attack as a nonsmoker.) Yet many people continue to smoke because they don't experience any noticeable physical problems. Others say, "The damage is done, so why quit now?" What many people fail to realize is that the risks from smoking *can* be lowered by reducing or, even better, by quitting the habit — even after many years of smoking.

The falloff in risk is dramatic. Even in those who have had a heart attack, risk of a second one will fall by about a third after 3 months, and by half after 2 years of quitting smoking.

STOP NOW

If you're a smoker and have *not* had a heart attack, quitting now can cut down your risk of heart attack to the level of a nonsmoker in as little time as a few months to a few years. There may still be damage to the lungs, but one of the major causes of heart disease will be eliminated. Over 6 times as many people die each year from heart disease as from lung cancer.

Even smokers with heart-related chest pain benefit when they quit smoking. After a few weeks, they usually see a drop in their heart rates and may show some improvement in electrocardiogram test results. Smoking also interferes with treatment for angina. Patients have seen less frequent episodes of angina after quitting smoking in as little as 6 to 8 weeks. In addition, their medication becomes more effective.

> *The best way to quit is to stop at once. Don't try to taper off.*

NICOTINE WITHDRAWAL

The active ingredient in tobacco is nicotine. Over years of smoking the body gets used to a certain level of nicotine. When you stop, you may experience mood or body changes, as follows:

- *Sluggishness, tiredness:* Due to lack of the nicotine stimulant, sleeplessness or dreams about smoking may occur.
- *Irritability, nervousness:* Exercise may help to alleviate these feelings.
- *Cough, dry mouth:* When you quit smoking, the lungs start kicking out mucus. The body will be producing less mucus, so the mouth may feel dry.
- *Hunger:* The urge for a cigarette may feel like a hunger pang. To deal with the urge, try drinking a glass of water.

Smoking-related diseases are such important causes of disability and premature death in developed countries that the control of cigarette smoking could do more to improve health and prolong life in these countries than any single action in the whole field of preventive medicine.

–World Health Organization

181

Cigarette smoking causes more premature deaths than automobile accidents, suicides, homicides, and AIDS combined.

–Michael Skeels
Oregon Health Division
(Oregon now requires that death certificates state whether tobacco use was a contributing factor.)

EXERCISE TO THE RESCUE

Along with joining a smoking cessation club and chewing nicotine gum, exercise may be the best way to eventually quit smoking. When you start an aerobic exercise program and pursue it regularly, you'll soon find that smoking and exercise don't mix. You get out of breath easily. Exercise can also be an alternative to eating and smoking, and will relieve irritability, encourage sound sleep, and ease depression during nicotine withdrawal.

TIPS FOR URGES

In addition to regular physical activity, there are several exercises that can reduce the urge to light up a smoke:

- Take 10 deep breaths and hold the last breath while you strike a match. Exhale slowly, blowing out the match. Pretend the match was a cigarette by crushing it out in an ashtray. Now immediately get busy on some work or activity.
- Take a brisk 5-minute walk for an energy boost.
- Squeeze a ball with your hand 20 to 40 times. This will keep your hands busy.

WEIGHT WATCHING

As you may know, many people who quit smoking gain weight. One reason is that calories aren't burned off as fast as before (nicotine is a stimulant and increases metabolism). More often, it's because new ex-smokers eat when they can't smoke, substituting food for cigarettes. You can help avoid those extra pounds by exercising regularly, drinking extra water (6 to 8 glasses a day), substituting low-calorie snacks such as popcorn, sugarless gum, and raw vegetables, and avoiding too much sugar. Weigh yourself every day. Don't let things get out of hand, but at the same time don't panic if you gain a few pounds.

ACCENTUATE THE POSITIVE

Remember to focus on the benefits. Once you stop smoking, your body and mind will feel better. You'll have more energy. You'll breathe easier. Best of all, you'll be proud of your accomplishment — it's tough to do! You'll have done a great thing for yourself and your future.

RECOMMENDED READING

The No-Nag, No-Guilt, Do-It-Your-Own-Way Guide to Quitting Smoking by Tom Ferguson, M.D., © 1988. Ballantine Books, New York, NY.

Stop Smoking Program Guide. American Cancer Society, New York, NY.

The Stop Smoking Book by Margaret K. McKean © 1987. Impact Publications, CA.

Smokers Anonymous. Check the white pages of your phone book.

STRESS

STRESS: THE BODY'S NATURAL RESPONSE TO STIMULI

Deadlines, traffic, long lines, noise, financial pressures, family worries, health concerns. We're all familiar with these common stresses of modern living and know it's important to relax. But what exactly is stress? And how does one relax?

Simply put, stress is the body's natural response to environmental and social stimuli. As external conditions change, the body's internal systems react to allow you to adapt to those changes and survive. These internal reactions are often called the "flight or fight response":

You're sitting in your most comfortable chair, engrossed in a novel when you hear a strange noise. Your senses come to attention. Where is that noise coming from? What is it? Your muscles tense, your heart is pounding, and you begin to perspire. You try to quiet your heavy breathing and notice you're gripping that novel like a weapon, ready to strike out. Should you fight or run and hide?

The flight or fight response is nature's way of protecting you in times of danger. That same response also helps you to meet challenges and achieve goals (for example, some tension before the "big game" helps a football team prepare mentally and physically to reach peak performance). The problem comes when stress is chronic and unrelieved. Your body is constantly on alert, and the protective changes brought on by stress can have a harmful effect on your mental and physical well-being, and even make you sick.

PHYSICAL CHANGES CAUSED BY STRESS

When your brain perceives a stress situation, it alerts the nerve centers in the spinal cord and the pituitary gland. The sympathetic and parasympathetic nerves stimulate your organs, and the pituitary gland signals the adrenal gland to produce adrenaline. The result:

- Heart rate increases and blood pressure rises.
- Respiration rate increases as oxygen consumption rises.
- Adrenaline, other hormones, and fatty acids are released into the bloodstream.
- The liver releases stored sugar.
- The muscles tense, particularly thighs, hips, back, shoulders, arms, and face.
- Blood flow to the digestive organs and extremities is constricted.
- Blood flow to the brain and major muscles increases.
- The body perspires to cool itself, since increased metabolism creates heat.

EFFECTS OF LONG-TERM STRESS

Every day your body reacts to 20 to 30 short-term stresses. Usually, there's time to recover in between, but sometimes these minor stresses are unrelenting. Other stresses (the illness of a relative, divorce, or worries about your career) may stay with you over long periods of time. When stress accumulates, your body and emotions feel the strain. Eventually, the brain's stimulation threshold actually drops, and even minor stresses cause a big physical reaction.

Doctors recognize a definite link between stress and heart disease, respiratory conditions like asthma, intestinal problems, and menstrual difficulties. Common headaches and migraines can be brought on or worsened by stress. Stress can also aggravate existing health problems. For example, it often exaggerates the symptoms of multiple sclerosis (MS) and diabetes. Emotional problems like anxiety and depression are frequently stress-related.

Evidence is growing that chronic stress wears down the immune system and increases your chance of getting sick. The constant presence of stress hormones in the bloodstream blunts the response of lymphocytes, weakening the body's ability to combat disease.

HOW EXERCISE RELIEVES STRESS

Stretching, moving, and lifting provide immediate relief from the physical symptoms of stress in several ways:

- Stretching and moving relax tense muscles.
- Exercise uses up the excess hormones, sugar, and fatty acids dumped into the bloodstream by the flight or fight response.
- During exercise, the body produces endorphins, neuroinhibitors that calm the stress response and create a peaceful, euphoric state (the "runner's high").
- Relaxation gained through exercise lasts many hours after the workout session.
- People who exercise and play sports are better at finding ways to relax and are more able to relax under pressure.

SPECIAL PROGRAMS

Try taking an exercise break instead of a coffee break at work. Include some exercise (even just a stroll) in your lunch hour. You'll find that some stretching and moving are much more refreshing, and ultimately more healthful, than ingesting caffeine and sugar! *(See pp. 33–40 for programs specially designed for exercising at work, on busy, stressful days, and while traveling.)* If you can exercise to relieve the physical and emotional symptoms of stress as they arise, you'll be calmer, more alert, and more comfortable, and you'll have less accumulated stress at the end of the day.

GOOD STRESS/BAD STRESS

Physical challenges like lifting weights or playing a tough game of tennis allow you to *feel* the stress reaction in your body and recognize it. Often in stressful situations, when your mind is absorbed by the problems at hand, you may not notice the reactions in your body — like higher blood pressure, faster heart rate, and tension in the muscles. But

PHYSICIAN, EXERCISE THY PATIENTS

A recent Gallup survey of 300 physicians found that 96% are concerned that people over age 40 do not get enough exercise, but 64% indicated they do not prescribe exercise because they lack the appropriate educational materials. If this is the case, we suggest doctors use this book as a guide. You can use the various programs in this book to prescribe exercise for your patients. And you can alter or vary the programs according to your patient's individual condition and needs.

RECOMMENDED READING

Fit Over 40 is a physician kit containing tearsheets, brochures, and other information about exercise for physicians to pass out to patients. The kit is assembled by the American College of Sports Medicine and Advil, and is distributed free to physicians. For information, write Advil Forum on Health Education, 1500 Broadway, 25th Floor, New York, NY 10036.

The Physician and Sportsmedicine magazine is in a class by itself with respect to fitness information for physicians. It is a monthly journal for sports medicine specialists, and keeps up with the latest in topics of practical application to specific training problems. Write McGraw-Hill, 4530 West 77th St., Minneapolis, MN 55435.

Sportsmedicine offers surveys of research literature and current knowledge in sports-related topics. Published 6 times annually by Adis Press International, Suite 830, Oxford Court Business Center, 982 Middletown Blvd., Langhorne, PA 10047.

Medicine and Science in Sports is published 6 times annually for the American College of Sports Medicine, 401 West Michigan St., Indianapolis, IN 46202.

The American Journal of Sports Medicine is published 6 times annually by Williams & Wilkins, 428 East Preston St., Baltimore, MD 21202.

Exercise and simple physical activity can help nearly all patients lead healthier lives, but the generic prescription must be tailored to fit each person's circumstances. "There is no magic bullet," says Harold W. Kohl III, MSPH, an epidemiologist with the Center for Aerobics Research in Dallas. "In fact, people who promote global exercise prescriptions — those very precise prescriptions for a broad range of people — are probably being irresponsible. Many physicians have discovered that a firm, but gentle, plug for exercise of any kind and amount can coax patients into routine physical activity."

–The Physician and Sportsmedicine

The Index of Stretches (p. 206) and the Index of Exercises (pp. 207–211) will be especially useful to doctors in designing exercise programs tailored to individual needs.

8 CHOOSING A GYM

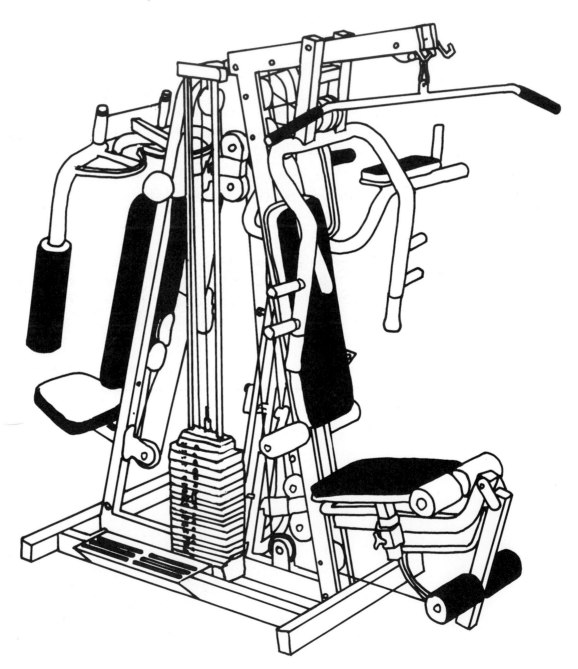

CHOOSING A GYM

HEALTH CLUBS

Health clubs differ from bodybuilding gyms in that they have less weight training equipment and are usually set up for general conditioning and socializing. A club is often a good place to start, with a variety of activities available and not as hardcore a weight training attitude as in the bodybuilding gyms. Also, as weight training becomes more popular, the clubs are constantly improving and adding equipment. Some of the larger clubs have a huge amount of equipment available. Watch out for hard-sell advertising, however — some of these clubs need a large membership to support high operating costs, and they can be overcrowded.

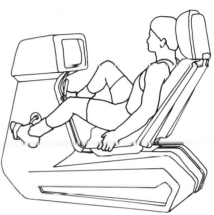

SCHOOL/YMCA WEIGHT ROOMS

School or YMCA gyms vary widely. Many large universities have excellent gyms for training athletes. Often school weight rooms are lively and full of enthusiastic and energetic students — it can be catching! In some gyms, there will be a lack of respect for equipment—plates scattered on the floor, nothing returned to its proper place. Sometimes broken equipment can't be fixed until the next year's school budget.

YMCA gyms have improved a lot in recent years in order to compete with private gyms. Even though they may not be as well equipped as some private gyms, they will probably have enough equipment for your general conditioning program. YMCA gyms are also a good place to work out when you're travelling.

BODYBUILDING GYMS

These are for serious weight training. They are usually well equipped with a variety of free weights and machines and often have qualified instructors who can advise you on your training. Here is what to look for:

- Condition of equipment and cleanliness. If the place is dirty, in need of repair or the weights are scattered around on the floor, it's a sign of poor management.
- Type of people training there. Do you feel comfortable around them?
- Management/instructors. Tell them what you want to do, your goals. Do they seem helpful?
- The emphasis of the gym. Is it compatible with your goals?

HOME GYMS

Exercising at home may not be a new concept but, today, exercise equipment for the home gym has become more accessible, attractive, and affordable. A home gym for total aerobic and resistance training can be assembled in an area as small as 100 square feet for under $1000. Or, at the other end of the scale, some people build special rooms in their homes, filled with computerized training equipment, for $15,000 or more.

Advantages of a Gym at Home

- You can work out any time of day or night.
- You save time — no travelling to a gym, no waiting for equipment.
- You can concentrate better, with no distractions.
- The whole family (and friends) can get involved.

Disadvantages of a Home Gym

- It may be hard to stay motivated when working out alone. A solution is to find a training partner — a family member or a friend. You make an appointment to meet for a workout and it's an incentive for both of you.
- A lot more equipment is available in a commercial gym.

Aerobic Equipment

The most popular and practical aerobic device for indoors is the stationary bike. Treadmills and stairclimbers are also widely used, but they are more expensive. Other widely used aerobic devices are rowing machines and cross-country ski machines. These machines all have the obvious advantage that they can be used indoors, at any time of day or night, even in the worst weather.

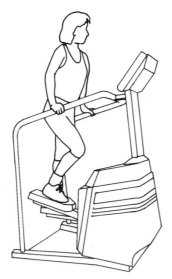
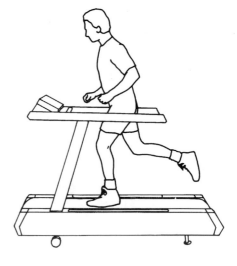

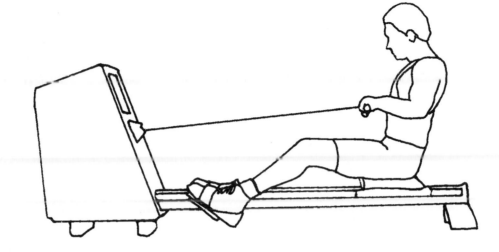

Picking the machine that is best for you is a matter of preference. Choose the equipment that simulates the activities you most enjoy. If you like walking, consider a treadmill or stairclimber. If you enjoy cycling, a stationary bicycle may be best.

Many people look upon the home gym as an opportunity to diversify their exercise programs. A rowing machine or cross-country ski machine can supplement your outdoor walking and cycling. Or an indoor bicycle can provide good cross-training for a jogging or running program.

An indoor alternative to buying an aerobic machine is to climb some stairs. If you live where there is a stairwell, walking up and down the steps for 5 to 10 minutes can provide an intense and effective aerobic workout. Or, if your building has only one story, you can actually get a workout on one or two steps — up-two-three, down-two-three. You'll be surprised at the results.

Strength Training Equipment

Equipment for exercising muscles can range from something as simple as barbells, dumbbells, and a bench to an elaborate multistation workout machine. If you're having trouble deciding what to buy, visit a gym, health club, or fitness store with a variety of equipment and try it all. See which equipment best suits your exercise needs. Investigate the different brands. Chances are that a well-run health club will have equipment of proven reliability.

Free Weights for the Home Gym

A home gym can be equipped quite inexpensively. Watch the papers for used equipment and check in fitness stores for the best deals.

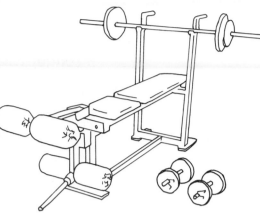

Here is a basic free weights setup for a hom

- One 60" x 1" barbell bar
- Two 14" x 1" dumbbell bars
- Four 10-lb plates
- Six 5-lb plates
- Collars for dumbbells
- One bench

Bench with leg extension attachment and adjustable back; standard 110 barbell/dumbbell set with two extra 25-lb plates.

In addition, it's a good idea to buy two 25-lb plates. There are deluxe versions and cheap versions. Get the best, as it will make your workouts more enjoyable. The plates with the machined holes are of higher quality that those with the cast holes. They slide on and off the bars smoothly and are a pleasure to handle. Chrome bars are the best and will last forever. We also recommend the chrome squeeze grip collars that make changing weights easy and quick.

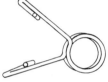

Another approach for the home gym is to get a multi-station machine, such as the Spirit Independence model shown at right. With a good machine like this, you can get a quick and satisfying workout. With the machine's weight stack, you can adjust weights by moving a pin, whereas with free weights you have to slide plates on and off the bars.

Strength Training with Homemade Equipment

- Use one-gallon milk jugs filled with different amounts of water as dumbbells.
- Make dumbbells with concrete in different sized tin cans, using steel water pipes for bars.

Strength Training with no Equipment

It's possible to get a decent workout in your home gym with no equipment at all. You merely follow a program of adequate stretching, calisthenics, a few pushups, and abdominal curls. The advantage, of course, is that no money is invested in equipment. The down side, however, is that without the gadgets, the variety of exercises is more limited, and home exercise can tend to get boring. *(See pp. 15–18, "The Program Before the Program," for 3 programs that utilize only your body weight for strength training workouts.)*

Sticking with It

Once you buy equipment, you'll want to stay motivated. You'll need to define your exercise goals and learn how to use the equipment properly. "Successful use of exercise equipment has to have 5 qualities," says Augie Nieto, president of Life Fitness, Inc. "It has to be motivational, injury-free, familiar in its biomechanical movement (like cycling and rowing), self-instructing and reliable."

Some gym owners hire consultants to work out an exercise program, coach them on new equipment, or provide encouragement. Indoor exercise needn't be boring. Attach a reading stand to your exercycle for reading while cycling, or watch the news or business report on TV while using a cross-country skiing machine. Watch TV or listen to the radio while lifting weights.

Take a little time to study the equipment you plan to buy, try it out first and see what feels right. You'll reap lasting returns.

APPENDICES

APPENDIX A

AMERICAN COLLEGE OF SPORTS MEDICINE FITNESS GUIDELINES

The American College of Sports Medicine (ACSM) is the largest sports medicine organization in the world. Since its inception in 1954, the ACSM has conducted activities regarding education, research, and information related to health and fitness, and is well known for publishing fitness guidelines.

The ACSM standards for fitness have gone through an evolution over the last two decades, reflecting the changing times. In 1978, the standards were quite high and, as the years passed, many exercise specialists came to realize that these levels of fitness were not necessary for good health. In addition, the high standards proved discouraging to most people.

If you are seeking a high level of fitness, the 1978 and 1990 goals are well worked-out guidelines. As we mentioned earlier in the book, once you have completed the 5 Basic Programs *(pp. 19–29)*, you should be in good enough shape to follow these guidelines.

However, for most people the latest (1993) revisions will be the most pertinent. They reflect a current major trend in the fitness world: A scaling back of over-ambitious goals with the emphasis on accumulating 30 minutes or so of *any* type of physical activity most days of the week.

A final note: Sedentary people have the most to gain from exercise programs. Those who go from no to moderate exercise realize dramatic health gains, whereas the fit who go from moderate to intense levels of exercise see only negligible improvements.

Following is a brief summary of the evolving guidelines.

THE 1978 GUIDELINES

In 1978, at the height of the 1970s fitness boom in America, the ACSM issued a position paper (intended for health professionals' guidance) entitled *The Recommended Quantity and Quality of Exercise for Developing and Maintaining Fitness in Healthy Adults*. The ACSM felt that the "increasing numbers of persons . . . becoming involved in endurance training activities" indicated a need for a statement on exercise. In the guidelines, fitness was equivalent to aerobic training. The paper set the standards for the:

- *Frequency*
- *Intensity*
- *Duration*
- *Mode* of aerobic exercise

In short, the paper recommended that a person should perform aerobic exercise 3 to 5 days per week for 15 to 60 minutes at a heart rate 60 to 90% of maximum. Aerobic exercise could include activities such as walking-hiking, running-jogging, cycling-bicycling, cross-country skiing, rope skipping, rowing, swimming, or skating.

Since that time, the ACSM guidelines have had a great influence on the type and amount of exercise prescribed by medical people and fitness-minded adults. These recommendations were quoted in thousands of fitness articles and books, and they influenced a new generation of physiology-wise fitness leaders.

THE REVISED 1990 GUIDELINES

Twelve years and much research later, the ACSM (in 1990) issued a revised and updated position paper. This time it was called *The Recommended Quantity and Quality of Exercise for Developing and Maintaining Cardiorespiratory and Muscular Fitness in Healthy Adults.*

The biggest news about the revised statement was that weight training was now being recommended as a major component in a total fitness program, whereas the 1978 statement had made only a passing reference to weight training — that it ". . . should not be considered as a means of training for developing maximum oxygen uptake (VO_2 max)."

Weight training was added to the recommendations because a 10-year study of master runners found that those who did no upper body training were losing upper body muscle mass. Those who continued aerobic training without upper body exercise maintained their VO_2 max, but lost 4.4 pounds of fat-free weight. On the other hand, those who included weight training in their fitness programs maintained a steady level of fat-free weight after 10 years of aging. The ACSM cited another 6 scientific studies prior to 1978 and 19 studies since 1978 in support of its recommendation for weight training.

There were also changes in the aerobic recommendations in the 1990 guidelines:

1. *Duration:* 20 to 60 minutes per session, rather than 15 to 60 minutes, as in 1978. The ACSM now recommends that you exercise aerobically for a longer time, but at moderate intensity. It was found that only those who are extremely fit can work at a high enough intensity to gain aerobic benefits from 15 minutes of training. Most people need to keep going for another 5 minutes to get the health benefits.

2. *Calculating exercise intensity:* An alternative method to the familiar pulse monitoring method was added in the new paper, called the *perceived exertion method (see below).*

SUMMARY OF THE 1990 ACSM GUIDELINES

Here is a summary of the main points of the 1990 guidelines:

1. *Cardiovascular Training*
   - *Frequency* of training: 3 to 5 days a week
   - *Intensity* of training: 60 to 90% of maximum heart rate, or 50 to 85% of VO_2 max or, as an alternative, the *perceived exertion method,* wherein you need not monitor your pulse during exercise. Here you make a subjective evaluation of how hard you're working — somewhere between "moderate" and "very heavy," which should correspond to 60 to 90% of heart rate maximum.

- *Duration* of training: 20 to 60 minutes of continuous aerobic activity. Lower intensity activity for a longer period of time is preferred to higher intensity for the nonathletic adult.
- *Mode* of activity: any activity that uses large muscle groups, can be maintained continuously, and is rhythmic and aerobic in nature, such as walking-hiking, running-jogging, cycling-bicycling, cross-country skiing, dancing, rope skipping, rowing, *stair-climbing*, swimming, skating and *various endurance game activities* (italics indicate additions to activities recommended in 1978).

2. *Resistance Training*
   - *Frequency* of training: at least 2 days a week
   - *Number* of exercises: a minimum of 8 to 10 exercises involving the major muscle groups
   - *Intensity* of training: a minimum of one set of 8 to 12 repetitions to near fatigue
   - *Mode* of activity: resistance training (weight training) is recommended, but traditional calisthenic exercises ". . . can still be effective in improving and maintaining strength."

3. *Stretching and Warm-up*

Although the ACSM does not give any specifics, it states: "An appropriate warm-up and cool-down, which would include flexibility exercises, is also recommended."

CONCLUSION

The ACSM concludes its paper by stating, "The important factor is to design a program for the individual to provide the proper amount of physical activity to attain maximal benefit at the lowest risk. Emphasis should be placed on factors that result in *permanent life-style change and encourage a lifetime of physical activity*" (italics ours).

It may be that the current low rate of participation is due in part to the public's perception that they must engage in vigorous, continuous exercise to reap health benefits. But actually, the scientific evidence shows that even moderate physical activity can also provide substantial health benefits.

—Russel L. Pate, Ph.D.
Past President, ACSM

NEW ACSM RECOMMENDATIONS, 1993

In 1993, the ACSM and the U.S. Centers for Disease Control and Prevention, in cooperation with the President's Council on Physical Fitness and Sports, convened a workshop on physical activity and health. Citing the fact that only 22% of American adults engage in physical activity at levels recommended for health benefits, the panel made new recommendations based on "an epidemic of inactivity" that was having a negative effect on the health of the nation and contributing substantially to the rising costs of health care.

Main Points of the 1993 Recommendations

"Every American adult should accumulate 30 minutes or more of moderate-intensity physical activity over the course of most days of the week. Incorporating more activity into the daily routine is an effective way to improve health. Activities that can contribute to the 30-minute total include walking up stairs (instead of using the elevator), gardening, raking leaves, dancing, or walking (part or all of the way) to or from work. The recommended 30 minutes of physical activity may also come from planned exercise or recreation, such as jogging, playing tennis, swimming, or cycling. One specific way to meet the standard is to walk 2 miles briskly.

"Because most adult Americans fail to meet this recommended level of moderate-intensity physical activity, almost all should strive to increase their participation in moderate or vigorous physical activity. Persons who currently do not engage in regular physical activity should begin by incorporating a few minutes of increased activity into their day, building up gradually to 30 minutes of additional physical activity. Regular participation in physical activities that develop and maintain muscular strength and joint flexibility is also recommended . . ."

RECOMMENDED READING

For further information on ACSM fitness guidelines write Public Information Department, ACSM, P.O. Box 1440, Indianapolis, IN 46206-1440.

APPENDIX B

THE FITNESS LIBRARY

AGING

Ageless Athletes: The Scientific Approach to Achieving High-Level Fitness and Counteracting the Effects of Aging by Richard A. Winett, Ph.D. (Contemporary Books, Chicago, IL, 1988)

> *"Health is a product of many interrelated factors such as diet, exercise, stress control, and interpersonal relationships."*

A highly technical, scientific approach to athletic performance. For those who like to chart progress this way, a set of principles is laid out for devising an individualized fitness program. A lot of attention is paid to the mind, learning how to monitor mood as well as the physical body. Positive thoughts, a calm, relaxed state, and focused concentration can enhance performance. Contains inspiring portraits of "masters", athletes who go on achieving maximum levels of fitness well into old age.

Smart Ways to Stay Young and Healthy by Bradley Gascoigne, M.D., and Julie Irwin (Ronin Publishing, Berkeley, CA, 1992)

> *"... discusses aerobics, power naps, back care, nutrition, immunizations, the Heimlich maneuver, cholesterol, finding a good doctor, breast exams, first aid, accidents, safe sex, substance abuse, smoking, stress, cancer, strokes, friendships, hobbies, meditation, affirmation, visualization, loving your work, and much more."*

Simply and concisely laid out in short, one- to two-page chapters, with recommendations and tips to guide you in conquering your addiction, stress, or ailment. Each chapter also lists additional resources for help and suggests further reading material. It seems that following all the advice in this book will guarantee your continued health and well-being.

We Live Too Short and Die Too Long: How to Achieve and Enjoy Your Natural 100-Year-Plus Life Span by Walter M. Bortz, M.D. (Bantam, New York, 1991)

> *"... Dr. Bortz sets out the essential, controllable elements of longevity and spells out effective, dynamic strategies to help you prevent premature death and add decades of active, satisfying life."*

The author puts forth the astonishing message that all of us are built to live well past a hundred years of age! This premise is backed by chapters of scientific evidence and his suggestions for basic healthy practices, which will increase our chances of living longer and more passionately.

FITNESS

Encyclopedia of Weight Training: Understanding the Scientific, Theoretical and Practical Basis of Weight Training by Robert D. Ward, P.E.D., and Paul E. Ward, P.E.D. (QPT Publications, Laguna Hills, CA, 1991)

"Weight training for general conditioning, sport and bodybuilding . . ."

A reference book that synthesizes scientific, theoretical, and practical information. Provides ample charts, tables, and scientific foundations for anyone engaged in coaching or teaching physical fitness, and using weight training as part of the program. The language and layout are academic, dry, and technical, but this is a great reference source. The book is likely to contain the practical information you're looking for. Contains programs for athletes or bodybuilders and information on nutrition.

Fitness Without Exercise: The Scientifically Proven Strategy for Achieving Maximum Health With Minimum Effort by Bryant A. Stamford, Ph.D., and Porter Shimer (Warner Books, New York, 1990)

"Grim details on the failure of the fitness movement."

Redefines fitness not as improved physical performance but rather as an increased feeling of health and well-being. Instead of intense aerobic exercise, the authors recommend establishing a prudent, low-fat, high-fiber diet, modest physical activity, and avoiding bad habits and stress. A fit diet is extremely important, and so is a "fit attitude" — the body and mind can work together to defend against such lifestyle-related diseases as heart attack, hypertension, and obesity. The Appendix features health-conscious recipes.

Getting Stronger: Weight Training for Men and Women by Bill Pearl and Gary T. Moran, Ph.D., (Shelter Publications, Bolinas, CA, 1986)

"The most complete book ever on weight training."

Bill Pearl is among the most respected champion bodybuilders of all time. In *Getting Stronger,* he has compiled his massive experience into easy-to-implement weight training programs for general conditioning, bodybuilding, or athletic training. He also offers his own conclusions on muscles, nutrition, injuries, and drugs, as well as a chapter on the history of resistance exercise.

Keys to the Inner Universe by Bill Pearl (Bill Pearl Enterprises, Phoenix, OR, 1982)

". . . complete information on 'weight-resistive exercise' for all who are interested in obtaining physical strength and health, increased power and ability in the performance of athletics, general physical fitness and conditioning, or advanced training techniques suitable for all body types."

Truly encyclopedic in scope and size, just doing curls with the book itself will tone your biceps! Besides detailed instructions on strengthening and toning each part of the body, Bill Pearl discusses "conduct becoming a champion," mental attitude, proper breathing, and nutrition.

Living with Exercise: Improving Your Health Through Moderate Physical Activity by Steven N. Blair, P.E.D. (American Health Publishing Company, Dallas, TX, 1991)

"Doing something is better than doing nothing."

The most important fitness book to come along in years — for the average person. Author Steven Blair recommends "lifestyle activities" as opposed to high levels of achievement in sports or other performance-oriented exercise regimens. By making increased activity a part of your daily routine, several times a day in short sessions, it's easy to include exercise as part of your busy schedule. Changing your attitude is significant, reflected in section titles like "Becoming Committed," "Overcoming Barriers" and "Planning for Change." A timely and excellent approach.

Maximum Muscular Fitness: Strength Training Without Equipment by Daniel P. Riley (Leisure Press, Champaign, IL, 1982)

"A revolutionary approach for developing strength through manual resistance exercises."

The exercises in this book use no dumbbells, barbells, or any other kind of traditional weight training equipment or paraphernalia. Resistance is provided by a training partner, and the advantages as well as disadvantages to this method are thoroughly discussed. Clear black and white photos make it seem easy, and the instructions are cautious and straightforward.

The New Fit or Fat by Covert Bailey (Houghton Mifflin, Boston, 1991)

"The ultimate cure for obesity is exercise."

The author contends that people are not overweight, they are overfat. Appropriate exercise will change your muscle chemistry to burn fat more efficiently. Increase the muscle enzymes that burn up the fat and carbohydrates you eat in order to improve metabolism. Aerobic exercise that demands uninterrupted output from your muscles for a minimum of twelve minutes is the way: steady, nonstop, at a comfortable pace.

Sitting on the Job: How to Survive the Stresses of Sitting Down to Work by Scott W. Donkin, D.C. (Houghton Mifflin, Boston, 1986)

> *"Create your best working environment by learning how to fit chair, lighting, and work space to increase comfort and productivity on the job."*

Addresses common physical complaints of the thousands of members of the clerical workforce who find themselves in a full-time sedentary job, and suggests ways to make it all better. From changing the physical setup of your office environment to changing your posture, breathing, habits, and attitude, this book will help you to "take the aching back out of your work."

Stretching by Bob Anderson (Shelter Publications, Bolinas, CA, 1980)

> *"Stretching helps keep your muscles flexible and ready for movement, improves performance, helps prevent injuries from physical activity and simply makes you feel good."*

With over 2 million copies sold, *Stretching* is just the best and most accessible book around. Contains over 1000 drawings and clear, concise instructions on the right and wrong way to stretch every part of the body, including stretches for everyday fitness as well as for running, tennis, racquetball, cycling, swimming, golf, and other sports. *Stretching* has been translated into 18 languages.

INJURIES

The Goodbye Back Pain Handbook: How to Treat and Prevent Back Pain by James A. Peterson, Ph.D., and James Wheeler, M.D. (Masters Press, Grand Rapids, MI, 1988)

> *"The human backbone is vital to the health and well-being of each person."*

After the anatomy lesson, the book categorizes the causes of back pain, and suggests ways to find the right doctor and therapies, and advice for daily living to prevent back pain in the first place. Introduces the Back Mate, an exercise apparatus that enables the hamstring and lower back muscles to be stretched effectively while the lower back and buttocks are strengthened safely. Done correctly, the exercises will bring immediate relief from pain.

The Human Body: Your Body and How It Works by Ruth D. Bruun, M.D., and Bertel Bruun, M.D. (Random House, New York, 1982)

> *". . . describes the interrelationships of all the working parts of your body."*

Full-color illustrations demonstrate beautifully the magnificent complexity of all the bones, organs, tissues and systems of the body. "No part of the human body works in isolation . . . To understand how the human body works, we must examine its systems one at a time. To understand the beauty and wonder of the human body, we must examine it as a whole. This book attempts to do both." An excellent book on anatomy and physiology for students — highly visual.

Listen to Your Pain: The Active Person's Guide to Understanding, Identifying and Treating Pain and Injury by Ben E. Benjamin, Ph.D. (Penguin Books, New York, 1984)

"Pain is a signal that something is wrong."

The best book available for sports injuries, whether from sports, an accident, or slow wear and tear. Tells you what the pain is, how you got it, how to evaluate it, and what your treatment choices are — from self-therapy to medical help and rehabilitation regimens. Presents highly technical material in a clear manner. Every pain has a cause. If you find it and treat it properly, you will get better. Catalogs injuries by body parts. A how-to guide to all the strains and stresses that can afflict active people.

Maggie's Back Book: Healing the Hurt in Your Lower Back by Maggie Lettvin (Houghton Mifflin, Boston, 1976)

"Our sitting habits, our fashions in clothing and furniture, the hard pavements of the city and the mental tensions that are reflected in general muscle tensions, all tend to make a sore back worse."

Rehabilitation requires mobilization and gradual strengthening of the tissues that support and move the spine — the soft tissues of the back and also the muscles of the abdomen and buttocks. How to identify the pain: what hurts, how much, what brings it on, then easing your way out, through stretching, exercise, painkillers, and new habits for everyday life. The best book available on back pain, and what to do about it yourself.

WALKING, RUNNING, CYCLING

Fitness Cycling by Chris Carmichael and Edmund R. Burke (Human Kinetics, Champaign, IL, 1994)

"...will help the intermediate to advanced cyclist avoid training ruts and continue progressing."

Contains 56 easy-to-use, color-coded cycling workouts — 45 on the road and 11 indoors — that provide a variety of exercise routines plus instructions for using the workouts to set up a personalized cycling program. The workouts are color coded according to degree of difficulty — green workouts are the easiest, red the hardest.

Galloway's Book on Running by Jeff Galloway (Shelter Publications, Bolinas, CA, 1984)

"Just when you thought that everything had been written about the simple act of running, along comes Jeff Galloway."

Still selling well almost 10 years since its first printing, *Galloway's Book on Running* provides all the information you need to make running a part of your exercise lifestyle, whether you want to run competitively or just around the block. There are unique training and racing programs and tips on form and willpower, preventing and treating injuries, food, and shoes. The best-selling running book in America by an ex-Olympian who knows how to transmit knowledge to average, as well as top-level runners.

Dr. James M. Rippe's Complete Book of Fitness Walking by James M. Rippe and Ann Ward (Prentice Hall Press, New York, NY, 1994)

"To reach your personal best, take a walk."

Scientific research shows that walking produces the same short-term training and long-term health benefits as any other aerobic sport, is easier on the joints and bones than running or aerobic dance, promotes weight loss and stronger bones, and helps lower blood pressure levels. Includes walking for women and people over 50, hiking, walking with weights, injury prevention, plus the complete Rockport Fitness Walking Test.

Walking Medicine: The Lifetime Guide to Preventive and Therapeutic Exercisewalking Programs by Gary Yanker and Kathy Burton (McGraw-Hill, New York, 1990)

"Gentle on the body and calming to the mind, walking symbolizes a moderate, balanced, active life-style."

Walking is the best natural remedy for a broad spectrum of illnesses, from life-threatening disorders such as arthritis and depression, to everyday problems, such as stress, lack of energy, and weight gain. It is easy, safe, inexpensive, and can be done almost anywhere. Routines and programs: helping with joint and back pain, calming your mind, making a healthier heart and stronger muscles, keeping you trim, and slowing the aging process. The routines are designed for different stages of your life, and for different body types and problems.

ABOUT THE AUTHORS

Bob Anderson is the world's most popular stretching authority. For almost 20 years, Bob has "preached the stretching gospel" all over the world. His book *Stretching* has sold over 2 million copies worldwide and has been translated into 18 languages (including two Chinese dialects).

Bob and his wife Jean self-published the first version of *Stretching* in a garage in Southern California in 1975. The drawings were done by Jean, based on photos she took of Bob doing the stretches. Their homemade book was modified and published by Shelter Publications in 1979 for general bookstore distribution and is now known by millions of people, from bookstore buyers to doctors, chiropractors, and exercise physiologists as the most accessible and useful book on the subject.

Today, Bob travels around the country, appearing at medical clinics, health conventions, training camps, and fitness centers. His appearances generally involve getting (himself and audience) down on the floor and doing a series of gentle stretches. All the while Bob talks about good health and the importance of keeping one's body strong and flexible and the heart and cardiovascular system in good shape.

Bob is fit and healthy these days, but it wasn't always so. In 1968, he was overweight (190 pounds — at 5'9") and out of shape. He began a personal fitness program that got him down to 135 pounds. Yet one day, while in a physical conditioning class in college, he found he couldn't reach much past his knee in a straight-legged sitting position. So Bob started stretching. He found he soon felt better and that stretching made his running and cycling easier.

Since that time, Bob has continued to practice what he preaches. He spends several hours each day running on the steep mountain trails above his house in Colorado and riding his mountain bike. He regularly runs the Catalina Island Marathon in Southern California, the 18-mile Imogen Pass mountain run in Telluride, Colorado, which goes up over a 13,000-foot-high ridge, and the Pikes Peak Marathon.

Though Bob works out long and hard each day, he knows that training like this is not for the average person. Through his travels, lectures, and workshops, he's kept in constant touch with people in all degrees of physical condition.

Bill Pearl is one of the greatest bodybuilders of all time. He is a former Mr. California, Mr. America, and four-time Mr. Universe. He was voted the World's Best Built Man in 1974 and called by *Sports Illustrated* ". . . the Sam Snead, Bill Tilden, and Gordie Howe of bodybuilding."

Bill began lifting weights at 11 years of age, and owned and managed world-renowned bodybuilding gyms in Southern California for over 30 years.

In the 1980s, Bill and his wife Judy (also a bodybuilder) self-produced a remarkable book, *Keys to the Inner Universe.* It is by far the most complete bodybuilding book ever written — 638 pages, weighs 5 pounds, and contains 1500 weightlifting exercises (86 for the chest, 193 for the biceps, etc.)

In 1986, Bill and Shelter Publications produced an entirely new book, intended for bodybuilders, serious athletes (with programs for 21 different sports) and also included conditioning programs for the average person. *Getting Stronger* has gone on to sell over 300,000 copies and is now the best-selling weight training book in America.

Like Bob Anderson, Bill is out on the road much of the year. These days he works for Life Fitness, manufacturers of the Lifecycle and the LifeCircuit line of electronic resistance weight training machines. He travels all over America and to Europe and Japan speaking to trainers, professionals, and amateurs interested in physical fitness.

Bill and Judy live on a ranch near Medford, Oregon. Behind their house is a barn filled with a complete line of both conventional and electronic weight training equipment. Bill is well known for his 6 days-a-week training routine. He gets up a 3 A.M., has a cup of tea, and stretches and warms up in his gym until 4:30, when his training partners arrive. Together, they train for about 2 ½ hours. Bill is over 60 years old and looks at least 10 years younger. He is known for his ability to transform his vast knowledge of fitness training into terms readily understandable to the average person.

Ed Burke has a master's degree from Ball State University in Indiana and a Ph.D. from Ohio State University. At Ball State, he worked with Dave Costill, the highly acclaimed director of the Human Performance Laboratory.

In the early 1970s, Ed had been a competitive cyclist for some years, riding in 25- to 100-mile road races. He saw that apparently no one (at least in the United States) had thought of applying scientific principles to cycling. So Ed began trying out some new concepts on himself and his cycling friends on the campus. Costill worked with them, doing interval and power work on exercycles in the lab, and Ed and his 5-man fraternity team went on to win their college race 2 years in a row.

Ed eventually went to work as Technical Director, then Director, of the Center for Science, Medicine and Technology at the U.S. Cycling Federation in Colorado Springs in the 1980s. During the 1984 Olympics in Los Angeles, the principles of exercise physiology as applied to cycling apparently paid off: on the very first day of the games, the U.S. team won 2 gold medals, the first cycling medals won by Americans in 72 years. The U.S. cyclists went on to win 3 golds, 3 silver, and 2 bronze medals in a sport previously dominated by European cyclists.

Ed met Bob Anderson in the mid-1980s. Ed was working in Texas for Spenco (manufacturer of insoles) at the time, and he went to Colorado to visit Bob. Bob's ideas on fitness made Ed realize he needed to make a change in his life and he moved to Colorado and started training with Bob in the mountains. Within 18 months, he dropped his resting heart rate to the 50s, lost 20 pounds, and achieved a long-time goal by running the Pikes Peak Marathon.

These days Ed and his wife Kathleen live in Colorado Springs and Ed is the director of the Exercise Science program at the University of Colorado at Colorado Springs.

INDEX OF STRETCHES

I. LOWER BACK, HIPS, GROIN, AND HAMSTRINGS   p. 78

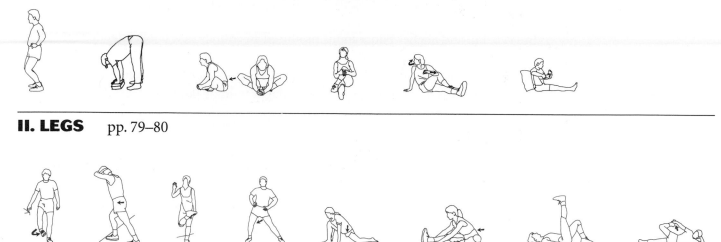

II. LEGS   pp. 79–80

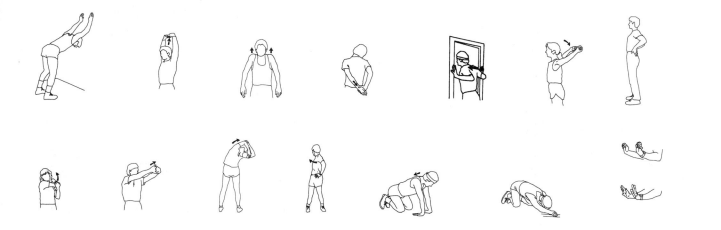

III. UPPER BODY: BACK, SHOULDERS, ARMS, AND HANDS   pp.81–82

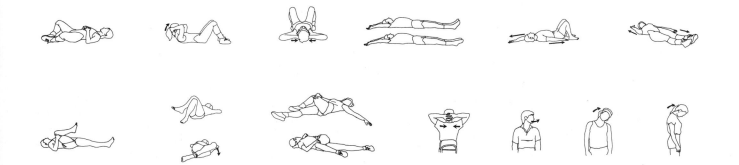

IV. BACK AND NECK   pp. 83–84

INDEX OF EXERCISES

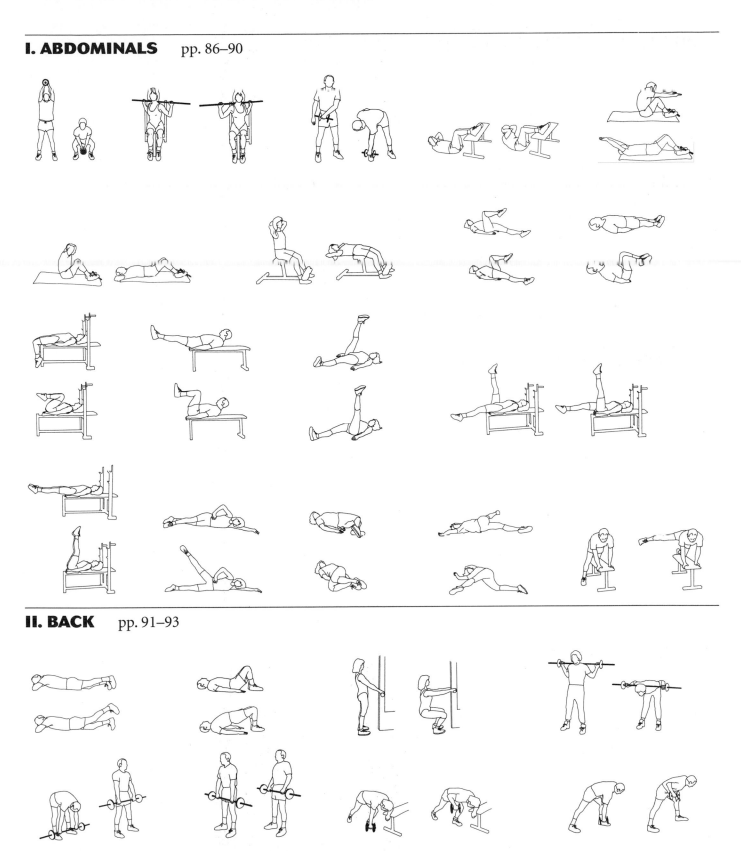

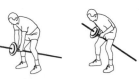

III. BICEPS   pp. 94–95

IV. CALVES   p. 96

V. CHEST   pp. 97–99

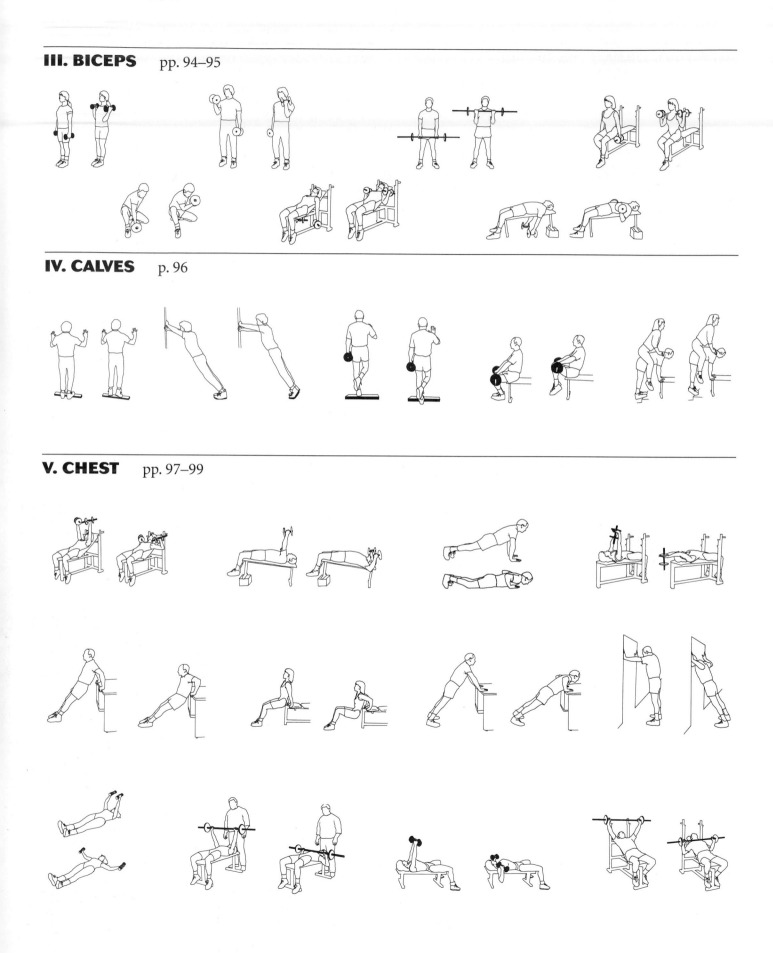

VI. SHOULDERS pp. 100–102

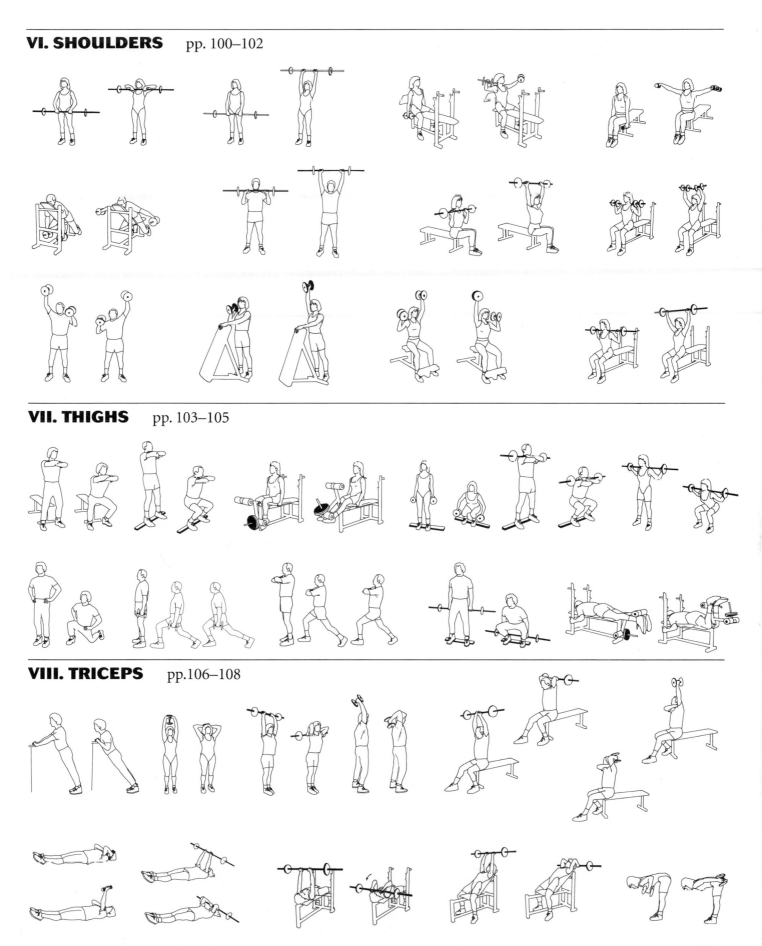

VII. THIGHS pp. 103–105

VIII. TRICEPS pp.106–108

Index

CREDITS

Editor
Lloyd Kahn

Contributing Editor
Stuart Kenter

Design
Janet Bollow

Production
Janet Bollow
Christina Reski
Rick Gordon

Typesetting
Christina Reski
Janet Bollow

First phase Project Manager
Marianne Rogoff

First phase editorial input
Marianne Rogoff
Charlotte Mayerson
Michael Rafferty

First phase design input
Suzanne Parks
David Wills

Cover design
Suzanne Parks
David Wills
Jean Anderson

Cover production
Rick Gordon
Suzanne Parks

Rendering, large-scale drawings
David Wills

Medical illustrations
Edna Indritz Steadman

Proofreading, Indexing
Frances Bowles

Models for drawings
Bob Anderson
Jean Anderson
Loyd Bell
Terry Cammicia
Paul Comish
Billy Cummings
Debra Gentile
Jody Matlock
Bill Pearl
Carol Roche
Rocky
Belinda Zell

Photography of models
Jean Anderson
Lloyd Kahn
Judy Pearl

Scans of drawings
Janet Bollow

Scanner
LaCie SilverScanner

Production hardware
Macintosh II FX

Programs
QuarkXpress 3.3
Adobe Photoshop 2.3.1
Adobe Illustrator 5.5
Adobe Streamline

Typefaces
Adobe Minion, Cosmos, Zapf Dingbats

Paper
60 lb. Pentair suede

Film
Marinstat Graphic Arts, Mill Valley, California

Printing
Courier Companies, Inc., Westford, Massachusets

Press Personnel, First Printing
Web Press Superintendents:
Dwight C. Woodward
Chuck Baker

Pressmen:
Roger Millette
Glen Kimball

Roll Tenders:
Mark Bray
George Rondeau

Press
Hantscho 4 Webb Offset

Special thanks to the following people who helped with this book in one way or another:
Howard Dillon
Dennis Hadley
Bridget Marmion
Joan Creed
Lesley Kahn
Eugene M. Schwarz
Bill Wright

MORE SHELTER FITNESS BOOKS

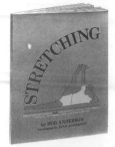

Stretching by Bob Anderson, illustrated by Jean Anderson
© 1980; 192 pp. paperback; ISBN 0–394–73874–8
$13.00

The classic book on stretching (over 2 million copies sold, in 25 languages). If you enjoy the stretching in *Getting in Shape,* this book covers the subject in detail, with routines for 20 sports as well as stretches to do while watching TV, for every day, for people over 50, for lower back pain, etc.

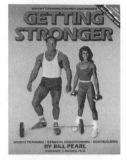

Getting Stronger by Bill Pearl and Gary T. Moran, Ph.D.
© 1986; 464 pp. paperback; ISBN 0–679–73269–1
$19.00

The most complete book on weight training ever. The logical next step if you want to progress beyond the weight training sections in Getting in Shape. Includes strength training for 21 different sports, three 45-minute workouts a week for general conditioning, as well as three levels of bodybuilding programs. The best-selling book on weight training in America

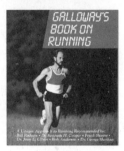

Galloway's Book on Running by Jeff Galloway
© 1984; 288 pp. paperback; ISBN 0394–72709–6
$13.00

Olympic runner Jeff Galloway shows how the same training principles used by elite runners apply to runners of all levels, explains his secrets for running better, his revolutionary ideas on stress and rest, tells beginners how to get started sensibly, and provides unique training charts for 10K races and marathons. State-of-the-art running.

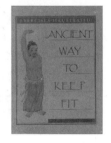

Ancient Way to Keep Fit by Zong Wu and Li Mao
© 1992; 224 pp. paperback; ISBN 0–679–41789–3
$20.00

From mainland China, this beautifully illustrated book contains 30 sets of exercises from ancient Chinese classical works. These Taoist-based "Chi Gung" movements predate Tai Chi and focus on increasing "chi" or life force energy. Some describe it as "internal martial arts," and consider it even more basic to health and fitness than cardiovascular exercise.

▶ To order any of these books, send the listed price, plus $3 postage and handling to:
Shelter Publications, Inc., P. O. Box 279, Bolinas, CA 94924. Write for free catalog.

▶ VISIT US ON THE WEB: **http://www.shelterpub.com/**

MORE FITNESS PRODUCTS FROM THE AUTHORS

Stretching: For information on a variety of stretching products, including wall charts, videos, body tools, etc., contact Stretching, Inc., P. O. Box 767, Palmer Lake, CO, 80133 or call toll free 800–333–1307.

Weight Training: For information on *Keys to the Inner Universe,* over 100 training charts and other weight lifting products, contact Bill Pearl Enterprises, Box 1080, Phoenix, OR, 97535 or call 503–535–3363.

Fitness Cycling: For books and charts on conditioning and training for cycling, contact Burke SportScience Communications, 3240 Wade Court, Colorado Springs, CO 80917.